The Butterfly Effect of the Vagus Nerve

Unlock Your Body's Self-Healing Potential to Overcome Your Migraines, Anxiety, Depression, and More Chronic Pain and Mental Health Challenges

Alex Locklear

Table of content:

Chapter 1: The Unsung Hero of Your Nervous System

Introduction to the vagus nerve and its functions

Have you ever thought about how your body knows what to do without you having to think about it? How your lungs breathe, your heart beats, and your stomach breaks down food? There's like an invisible director in charge of the symphony of life inside you. Yes, there is!

This nerve is known as the vagus nerve.

Out of the twelve nerves that start in your brain, the vagus nerve is the longest and most complicated. To reach almost every major function in your body, this nerve spreads out like a network of roots. It's a two-way street that lets your brain and organs talk to each other. It affects everything from your mood and immune system to your heart rate and nutrition.

The vagus nerve is in charge of your body's "rest and digest" team. It's part of the parasympathetic nervous system, which is in charge of making your body feel better when it's under stress or danger. You're more likely to feel calm, happy, and healthy when your vagus nerve is healthy. But if it's not working right, you may be more likely to have health issues like anxiety, sadness, chronic pain, and more.

The good news is that you can train your vagus nerve just like you train your muscles. You can open a whole new level of health and wellness by learning how your body's natural healing power works and how to stimulate it in a simple way.

It's interesting to learn more about the vagus nerve and what it does. We will talk about how it impacts your brain, heart, lungs, gut, and immune system. You'll learn how important it is for dealing with stress, lowering inflammation, and making you feel calm. You will also discover how to use the power of your vagus nerve to deal with chronic pain, stress, sadness, and other health issues.

Are you ready to start this exciting trip to learn more about yourself? Let's figure out what the vagus nerve does and let your body heal itself in amazing ways. The Vagus Nerve is the main way your body talks to itself. The vagus nerve links your brain to your heart, lungs, gut, and other parts of your body. It's like a complicated web of wires. It sends and receives messages, moving information between your brain and organs and back again. For your body to stay balanced and in harmony, this two-way exchange is very important. For instance, when you're nervous or stressed, your brain tells your heart to beat faster through the vagus nerve. Your vagus nerve also sends signals from your heart to your brain. These signals tell your brain about your heart rate and other body processes. This feedback loop lets your brain change how it reacts and keep things in balance.

The vagus nerve is also very important for digestion. There is more stomach gas and enzymes when you eat this. These are needed to break down food. It also controls how food moves through your digestive system, making sure it's broken down and absorbed properly. How Your Immune System Works and the Vagus Nerve Did you know that the vagus nerve helps your defense system? It's real! Inflammation is a normal reaction to injury or infection, and the vagus nerve helps keep it in check. Although some inflammation is needed for recovery, too much of it can be bad and lead to long-term illnesses.

By releasing chemicals that reduce inflammation, the vagus nerve helps to keep it in check. It also talks to your immune cells and helps them work together to fight off illness or damage. The vagus nerve is linked to the immune system, which is one reason why stimulating the vagus nerve may help treat autoimmune diseases like rheumatoid arthritis and inflammatory gut disease.

What the Vagus Nerve Does for Your Mind

When it comes to your mental health, the vagus nerve is just as important as it is for your physical health. Keeping your mood stable, anxiety, and sadness have all been linked to it. When your vagus nerve works well, you're more likely to be happy, calm, and relaxed. But if it's not working right, you might be more likely to get anxiety, depression, and other mood illnesses. Researchers have found that stimulating the vagus nerve can help people who are depressed and anxious feel better. The FDA has approved vagus nerve stimulation therapy as a way to treat depression that hasn't responded to other treatments. This therapy includes implanting a device that sends electrical impulses to the vagus nerve. To activate your vagus nerve, you don't have to have surgery, though.

A lot of easy things you can do at home, like yoga, meditation, and deep breathing exercises, can help your vagus nerve work better and make you feel better.

A part of the autonomic nervous system (ANS) played by the vagus nerve

The vagus nerve does not work by itself. It's an important part of your nervous system as a whole, especially the autonomic nerve system (ANS). By understanding this link, you'll get a better idea of how deeply the vagus nerve affects your health.

The autonomic nervous system is like the GPS for your body.
You can think of the ANS as the boss of your body. It controls all the important things you don't even think about, like your heartbeat, breathing, digestion, and even the small changes in the size of your blood vessels. There are two main parts to the ANS:

Also known as the "fight-or-flight" system, the sympathetic nervous system. It gets your body ready for danger and worry. Your breathing gets faster, your heart beats faster, and your stomach slows down. Even though this reaction is necessary for survival, an SNS that is always on can cause long-term health problems. This is your "rest and digest" system, the parasympathetic nervous system (PNS). In contrast to SNS, it calms you down and helps your body heal and grow back. The vagus nerve is the most important nerve in the PNS because it communicates with the rest of the body.

The vagus nerve: a calm conductor

People often compare the vagus nerve to the director of an orchestra. It tells your body to slow down your heart rate, breathe more deeply, and digest food better when it's busy. This is what makes you feel calm and at ease after a nice meal or some yoga.

But the vagus nerve has effects that go far beyond making you feel calm. It is an important part of keeping your feelings and mind in check. Feelings of peace, happiness, and social connection are more likely to happen when your vagus nerve is toned and sensitive. To Keep Things in Balance: Vagal Tone and Resilience Your vagus nerve's strength and response are called its "vagal tone." Having a high vagal tone is linked to many benefits, such as:

• Lessened stress and sadness

• Better health for the heart

• Better ability to handle stress

• Better stomach health

• Less congestion

On the other hand, low vagal tone is linked to many health issues, varying from constant pain to digestive issues. It's good to know that vagal tone can change. You can make it better by doing things that activate and strengthen the vagus nerve.

How to Use the Vagus Nerve's Power

This book will talk about a lot of different ways to improve vagal tone and use your nervous system's ability to fix itself. You will learn how to use awareness, movement, breathing exercises, and even social interaction to stimulate your vagus nerve and make your body and mind feel better all   over.
Remember that the vagus nerve is more than just a nerve. It's a way to be strong, healthy, and have a life with less pain and more joy. Knowing what part it plays in the autonomic nervous system is the first thing that will help you use its transformative power.

There is more than one path in the vagus nerve. It's more like a huge network of roads that connect your brain to almost all of your body's major organs. It's like the freeway of your body; it sends and receives important messages to keep things in balance. A healthy vagus nerve keeps your body working at its best, just like a well-kept road system keeps traffic moving smoothly.

The control center of your brain

The medulla oblongata in the brainstem is where our trip starts. This part of the body controls important things like breathing, heart rate, and nutrition. The vagus nerve starts here and spreads out like a tree with roots firmly planted in the brain.

A Face-to-Face Link

Your face is the first thing that this highway hits. You can feel the vagus nerve in your eyes, ears, mouth, and throat.

Because of this, stimulating these areas by singing, gargling, or even splashing cold water on your face can turn on the vagus nerve and make it work to calm you down.

The Neck's Important Crossroads

The vagus nerve runs along major blood vessels in your neck and links to your vocal cords and the muscles that help you swallow. This link is important for speech and may be involved in conditions like problems with the vocal cords and swallowing issues.

From the Heart

The heart is one of the most important nerves that the vagus nerve connects to. It cools your heart rate down so you can save energy when you're not working out. This is why workouts that make you breathe deeply can help lower your blood pressure and heart rate.

The Gut-Brain Axis

It goes on past your heart and into your neck. It keeps going until it gets to your digestive system, where it is very important for gut health. It tells your stomach and intestines what to do, which can change nutrition, the way your gut moves, and even your immune system. Because of how strong this link is, scientists often call it the gut-brain axis. Having a healthy vagus nerve can help lower inflammation in the gut, ease the symptoms of irritable bowel syndrome (IBS), and even make you feel better.

Past the Gut

The vagus nerve does more than that, though. It's also linked to your pancreas, kidneys, liver, and spleen. In other words, it helps control your blood sugar, remove toxins from your body, and make hormones that impact your mood and stress reaction.

The Nerve That Wanders

As the vagus nerve runs through the body, it's no surprise that it's called the "wandering nerve." It really does wander from your brain to your organs, connecting them and changing how they work. Because of its complex web of links, stimulating the vagus nerve can have such a big effect on your health and well-being as a whole.

How to Use the Vagus Nerve's Power

Figuring out the vagus nerve's paths and links is like finding a secret map to your body's ability to fix itself. To use this nerve's healing power, do simple things like deep breathing, singing, gargling, or even mindful eating. These can help lower stress, improve digestion, ease pain, and improve your mood. Your body has a built-in way to heal itself and ease stress called the vagus nerve. When you turn it on, you're basically opening the door to your body's natural pharmacy. It releases a chain of good chemicals that help you relax, reduce inflammation, and improve your overall health.

The vagus nerve is like the director of the orchestra that is your body. When everything is working right, your organs are like musicians who all play together in perfect harmony, making a beautiful symphony of health and energy. But if the vagus nerve is out of tune, the music is off, which can cause a number of health issues. You can take charge of your health and let your body's natural ability to heal and grow shine through if you understand and care for this important nerve. Now is the time to make the vagus nerve your friend on your way to better health.

The "fight or flight" response is an old way to stay alive. Let's start with a situation that you may already know all too well. Picture yourself going down a dark street by yourself late at night. Your heart starts beating fast when you hear footsteps behind you. Your muscles tense up, your breath speeds up, and you feel a rush of energy. Your body's "fight or flight" response is activating. This is a survival strategy that has been built in since we lived in caves.

Our sympathetic nerve system takes over when we sense a threat, whether it's real or not. In a way, it's like a quick response team getting our bodies ready to either fight or run away from danger. Our pupils get bigger to help us see better, our heart rate and blood pressure go up so that muscles get more oxygen and nutrients, and our stomach slows down so that our bodies can use their energy for more   important   tasks.
"Fight or flight" is an important reaction that helps us stay

alive in emergencies, but it's not supposed to be a permanent state of mind. If we stay in this high-alert state all the time, it can be terrible for our health and cause stress, worry, and a lot of different illnesses. The "Rest and Digest" Response is your body's way of healing itself.

This is where the "rest and digest" reaction comes in. It's the opposite of "fight or flight," a deep state of rest and healing. When we feel safe, our parasympathetic nervous system takes over. It lowers our blood pressure, slows down our heart rate, and helps our bodies digest food. It's like pressing the "reset" button on our bodies, which gives us the chance to get our energy back.

How does the vagus nerve fit into all of this? In fact, it's what makes the parasympathetic nervous system work, which makes our bodies feel calm. When the vagus nerve is stimulated, it tells our organs to calm down and rest. This is why deep breathing routines, meditation, and other forms of relaxation can help lower stress and improve health in general.

How to Use the Power of the Vagus Nerve to Find Balance

To be healthy, you need to find a good mix between your "fight or flight" and "rest and digest" responses. We need to be able to deal with problems when they happen, but we also need to be able to unwind and recharge so that stress doesn't get the best of us. The vagus nerve can make a big difference here. Through different methods, we can learn to activate our vagus nerve and make it easier for our bodies to go into "rest and digest" mode, even when things are tough. This can make us less anxious, help us sleep better, strengthen our immune systems, and make us stronger overall.

It's helpful to think of the vagus nerve as a light switch for your nervous system. By increasing the activity of the vagus nerve, you can turn down the "fight or flight" reaction and turn up the "rest and digest" response. This not only helps with the symptoms of chronic stress, but it also lets your body heal itself.

Your secret weapon for getting rid of chronic pain and mental health problems is the vagus nerve. A lot of different long-term conditions can be helped by stimulating the vagus nerve. These include migraines, anxiety, sadness, irritable bowel syndrome (IBS), and even long-term pain. A natural cure that can help you take back control of your health and well-being is like having a secret tool in your back pocket.

We'll look at different ways to stimulate your vagus nerve and use its healing power in the next few chapters. We'll talk about the science behind these techniques, give you tips on how to use them in your daily life, and share inspiring stories of people who have used vagus nerve stimulation to solve long-term health problems.

Remember that your body has a wonderful way of fixing itself, and the vagus nerve is the key to using it. You can lower your stress, boost your mood, and improve your health and well-being as a whole by learning how to trigger this powerful nerve. Let's go on this trip together and find out how the vagus nerve can change your life.

Chapter 2: The Vagus Nerve and Your Health

How the Vagus Nerve Affects Your Mind and Body
The Vagus Nerve is the main way your body talks to itself. The vagus nerve is like a superhighway for information; it sends messages all the time between your brain and the rest of your body. Your heart rate, digestion, mood, and immune reaction are just some of the things that it can send and receive. This exchange is very important for keeping your system in balance and harmony.

An Orchestra of Health and Happiness: The Vagus Nerve and Your Health

First, let's talk about how the vagus nerve controls your health. Another name for this nerve is the parasympathetic nervous system. It is an important part of the "rest and digest" system. The vagus nerve sets off a chain of relaxing reactions when it is activated. Your stomach gets better, your blood pressure goes down, and your heart rate slows down. For the most part, the vagus nerve helps your body heal and recharge.

But the vagus nerve does a lot more than just make you feel calm. It is very important for controlling inflammation, which is a process at the root of many long-term illnesses. Studies have shown that stimulating the vagus nerve can lower inflammation in the body. This could help people with rheumatoid arthritis and inflammatory gut disease.

It also talks to your gut, which is called your "second

brain." Scientists think this link is so strong that it affects everything from your mood to how well you digest food. Are you used to getting butterflies before a big event? That's the vagus nerve at work! Taking care of your vagus nerve can help your gut feel better, which will make you happy.

The Vagus Nerve and Mental Health: A Way to Get Strong Emotionally

Finally, let us talk about the interesting link between the vagus nerve and mental health. This nerve affects more than just our physical health; it also has a big effect on how we feel. Researchers have found that a healthy vagus nerve is linked to a better mood, less worry, and a stronger ability to handle stress. How does this work? The importance of the vagus nerve in controlling the stress response is one idea.

The "fight or flight" reaction is set off by our sympathetic nervous system when we sense danger.

Stress can put us in this high state for a long time, even though this response is necessary for survival. As a brake, the vagus nerve helps us calm down and get back on balance.

Neurotransmitters, such as serotonin and GABA, which are known to affect mood, also work with the vagus nerve. By stimulating the vagus nerve, we can get these chemicals that make us feel good to come out, which will make us feel better overall.

The Power of Vagus Nerve Stimulation in Real Life

The effects of the vagus nerve are not just ideas; they are based on study and examples from real life. As an example, Sarah was a woman who had a lot of trouble with worry. She was able to get back in charge of her life and greatly lower her anxiety levels by using a combination of vagus nerve stimulation techniques, such as deep breathing exercises and being exposed to cold air.

Vagus nerve stimulation has also shown promise as a way to treat sadness, PTSD, and even migraines. Even though more study needs to be done, these results give people with these difficult conditions some hope.

How to Use Your Vagus Nerve's Power

The great thing about the vagus nerve is that you can change how it works. You can calm your vagus nerve and get all of its health benefits by doing easy things like deep breathing, yoga, meditation, or even singing. We'll talk about these methods in more depth in later chapters, giving you a set of tools to improve the function of your vagus nerve.

Don't forget that your body has a great ability to fix itself, and the vagus nerve is a key part of that ability. You can improve your physical and mental health and live a more vibrant and satisfying life by taking care of this powerful nerve.

How the activity of the vagus nerve is linked to long-term conditions like migraines, anxiety, depression, and more

Our health is closely linked to the vagus nerve, which we've learned about in this chapter. But the story doesn't end there. The vagus nerve is not just a spectator, as you now know; it actively shapes how we feel when we are healthy or sick. We've already talked about how it affects general health, but now we'll talk about something even more important: how it's linked to chronic conditions like migraines, anxiety, and sadness that affect millions of people around the world.

The vagus nerve is like the conductor of a big orchestra, with each instrument reflecting a different part of your health. When the conductor keeps the rhythm steady, the music flows easily, providing balance and harmony. But if the director slips up, the music stops playing together, which causes chaos and discord.

The same thing is true for your body. According to research, problems with the vagus nerve can make a number of long-term diseases worse. Studies have shown that people who get headaches have lower vagal tone, which means their vagus nerve isn't working as well as it should. For some people, this can make them more sensitive to pain and more likely to have migraines.

Anxiety and sadness, those lingering clouds that cover so many lives, are also linked to problems with the vagus nerve. Your stress response system goes into action when your vagal tone is low. This makes it harder to relax and deal with the problems that come up in life. This can make you feel anxious and hopeless, which can keep you stuck in a cycle of mental pain.

The good news is that the vagus nerve affects long-term symptoms in both directions. These situations can get worse when vagal tone is low, but they can get better when vagal tone is high. This is where the vagus nerve's real power lies: it can help your body heal itself and give you long-lasting comfort.

You can think of it as retuning the music in your body. By making your vagus nerve stronger, you're basically helping the conductor get back in charge, which will make your health's songs sound better again. This can lead to fewer migraines, less stress, and a better view on life.

Allow me to tell you a story to make this point clear. Sarah, a lively woman in her 40s, had been dealing with headaches for many years. She had tried many medicines and therapies, but nothing seemed to help her in the long term. She came across the idea of vagus nerve stimulation one day and decided to give it a try. Sarah started doing easy vagus nerve exercises every day, like taking deep breaths and immersing herself in cold water. She didn't see much of a change at first, but she kept going because she believed in the process. Over time, she started to have fewer migraines, and her general health got better. Sarah was no longer just dealing with her headaches; she was taking charge of her health again.

Stories like Sarah's are not rare occurrences. Using the power of their vagus nerve has helped a huge number of people with long-term diseases. They've not only gotten better by making simple changes to their lifestyle and using targeted vagal stimulation methods, but they've also gotten rid of their symptoms. The great thing about vagus nerve activation is that anyone can do it. You don't need to have expensive tools or special training. For a short time every day, you can start to strengthen your vagus nerve and let your body heal itself naturally.

In the next chapter, we'll talk more about how these ideas can be used in real life. We'll look at specific vagus nerve exercises and changes you can make to your daily practice. For now, though, let the fact that you are the one who can fix yourself sink in. Accept the power of your vagus nerve and start the path to a healthier, happy you.

What Stress and Trauma Do to the Vagus Nerve

We've talked about how the vagus nerve is very important to our health because it controls the parasympathetic nervous system, which is like the "rest and digest" reaction to our "fight or flight" response. Now, let's talk about how stress and trauma can throw this delicate balance off, causing a wide range of health problems, such as the migraines, anxiety, sadness, and long-term pain that so many of us deal with.

You can think of the vagus nerve as a highway that runs from your brain to your body's main organs. Your body works best when this highway is clear and traffic moves quickly. But when stress and trauma get in the way of this route, communication breaks down. This can lead to a wide range of physical and mental health problems. Our sympathetic nervous system, or "fight or flight" mode, can be set off by different kinds of stress, such as short-term, long-term, or even the effects of a traumatic event. While this reaction is necessary to stay alive in an emergency, keeping it going for too long can damage our vagus nerve. It's hard for the vagus nerve to keep our bodies functioning normally when we're constantly on high alert. This can show up as stomach issues, a racing heart, trouble sleeping, and a weaker immune system.

Whether it's a single stressful event or ongoing pain, trauma can leave a deeper mark on our vagus nerve. Studies have shown that people who have been through a traumatic event often have lower vagal tone, which means their vagus nerve isn't working as well as it should. This can cause long-lasting inflammation, a stronger response to stress, and a heightened awareness of pain. The painful event seems to get "stuck" in the body, setting off the vagus nerve even when there isn't a threat at hand.

But here's the good news: our bodies are very strong, and the vagus nerve is no different. Even though trauma and worry can make it less effective, we have the power to heal and restore this important link. A skilled gardener can bring a plant back to health, and the same is true for us. There are many tools and techniques we can use to calm and balance our vagus nerve.

The breath is one of the most important tools we have. The vagus nerve is activated when you breathe deeply and slowly. It tells your brain and body that it is safe. It's like a saying "All is well" that calms you down. Breathing exercises like diaphragmatic breathing, alternate nostril breathing, and even just being aware of your breath can have a big effect on vagal tone.

Moving your body is another powerful way to stimulate the vagus nerve.

Whether you do easy yoga, tai chi, or a fast walk in the park, being active can improve vagal tone and release endorphins, which are chemicals that make you feel good and fight stress. The vagus nerve can be stimulated and relaxation can happen by doing easy things like humming or stretching.

Practicing good feelings like joy, gratitude, and kindness can also have a direct effect on vagal tone.

When we think about the good things in our lives, our vagus nerve sends messages to the rest of our bodies that we are healthy. Writing in a journal, meditating, and spending time with loved ones are all good ways to feel better and help the vagus nerve do its job of controlling our feelings.

This nerve is also affected by what you eat. Eating lots of healthy fats, fruits, and veggies that are low in inflammation can help vagal tone. On the other hand, processed foods, sugar, and caffeine can make it worse. The vagus nerve and gut health are closely linked, so eating fermented foods and probiotics can help the gut bacteria and vagus function in a roundabout way.

Getting in touch with other people is another important part of vagus nerve healing. Oxytocin is a hormone that is released when you interact with other people. It improves vagal tone and makes you feel connected and trusting. Getting together with other people, like seeing family and friends, joining a support group, or just petting your pet, can help you deal with stress and trauma.

Don't forget that healing is a process that is different for everyone. Try out different methods until you find the one that works best for you. By taking care of your vagus nerve and focusing on mental peace, you can help your body heal and grow naturally.

In the next chapter, we'll talk about some useful ways to stimulate the vagus nerve and make it work better. You'll learn specific exercises, breathing techniques, and changes to your lifestyle that can help you use your vagus nerve's power to get better health and live a longer, healthier life.

A link between the gut and the brain called the vagus nerve is part of your second brain.

Have you ever had a "gut feeling" or felt like you had "butterflies" in your stomach when you were scared? These aren't just words that mean something. They show that your gut and brain are strongly connected, and the powerful vagus nerve plays a big role in that link. The gut-brain axis is a two-way communication path where your gut, which is sometimes called your "second brain," and your brain talk to each other all the time. Everything about your health is affected by this dynamic interaction, from your immune system and general health to your digestion and mood. The vagus nerve is at the center of it all.

The vagus nerve connects two worlds.

The vagus nerve is like a busy freeway. It's made up of a huge network of nerve fibers that carry messages from your gut to your brain. The nerve starts in the brainstem and goes through the neck, chest, and belly, connecting to organs like the heart, lungs, and most importantly, the digestive system. It is the longest nerve in the head. A very important part of the parasympathetic nervous system, which is also known as the "rest and digest" system, is this nerve. It helps your body relax after being stressed, slows down your heart rate, and digests food better. But it does a lot more than just these simple things.

The Second Brain Does More Than Digest Food

There are a lot of neurons, neurotransmitters, and bacteria in your gut, so it's not just a place where food is broken down. It is thought that your gut has about the same number of neurons as your spinal cord. The enteric nervous system (ENS) is made up of these neurons. It is a complicated network that can work without the brain, which is why it is sometimes called "the second brain." The ENS is in charge of digestion, your immune system, hormone production, and even your mood.

The gut microbiome, which is made up of the trillions of bacteria that live in your digestive system, has been shown to affect many things, from your stress response and anxiety levels to your risk of depression and other mental health problems.

How the gut-brain axis works: a two-way street

Communication between your gut and brain goes both ways; information is always going back and forth along the vagus nerve. For example, when you eat, your gut tells your brain about the nutrients it's getting. This helps keep your energy and hunger levels in check. It's not just about food, though. Your gut also tells you about its general health, such as any pain, stress, or inflammation.

These messages can cause changes in your brain that can affect your mood, your ability to think and remember things, and even how you feel pain. In turn, your brain sends messages back to your gut, which changes how it works and what kinds of bacteria live there. The gut-brain axis stays balanced thanks to this ongoing communication, which is good for your health and well-being as a whole.

The Link Between Your Gut and Brain and Your Health

More and more studies show that the gut-brain link has a big effect on many parts of health. Studies have found links between gut health and many health problems, such as • Mental Health: The gut microbiome has been linked to a number of mental health problems, such as autism, depression, and worry. Some probiotics, or good bacteria, have been shown in studies to improve happiness and lower anxiety in some people.

• Digestive Health: The gut-brain link is very important for digestive health. It affects everything from bowel movements and nutrient absorption to irritable bowel syndrome (IBS).

• Immune Function: For a strong immune system, you need a good gut microbiome. A lot of your immune cells live in your gut, and problems with the bacteria in your gut can make you more likely to get infections and autoimmune diseases.

• Long-Term Pain: Studies show that the link between the gut and brain may be important in conditions like fibromyalgia and headaches that cause long-term pain.

Some studies have shown that taking care of your gut can help you feel better and have less pain.

How to Take Care of Your Gut-Brain Link

How then can you keep this strong bond going and let your body heal itself? Here are some ideas: • Eat a healthy diet. Fiber-rich foods, fruits, veggies, and fermented foods can help keep your gut microbiome healthy and make it easier for your gut and brain to talk to each other.

• Deal with stress: Long-term stress can mess up the connection between your gut and brain. To deal with worry in a healthy way, do things like exercise, meditate, or spend time in nature.

• Think about probiotics. These are good bacteria that can help balance your gut microbiome and make interactions between your gut and brain better. Check with your doctor to see if probiotics are a good idea for you.

• Make sleep a priority. Sleep is important for your gut-brain axis health and for your general health. Try to get between 7 and 8 hours of sleep each night.

New research on vagus nerve stimulation (VNS) shows that it may be a good way to treat a number of conditions, such as depression, epilepsy, and even inflammatory bowel disease. Electrical impulses are used to stimulate the vagus nerve during VNS. This can help control how it works and make contact between the gut and brain better.

You can find a powerful way to heal and be healthy by learning and taking care of the connection between your gut and brain. Remember that your gut is more than just a place where food is broken down; it plays a big role in your health and happiness as a whole.

Chapter 3: Signs of a Dysregulated Vagus Nerve

Common Symptoms of Low Vagal Tone

Today, we're going to talk about the signs that your vagus nerve may not be working as well as it should. Remember that the vagus nerve controls many body processes like a conductor for a symphony. The orchestra can sound a little off when one instrument is out of tune.

When this conductor has a low vagal tone, it means it isn't leading with its normal gusto. Your body's "rest and digest" mode is turned down by this. This can show up in many forms, from physical illnesses to mental problems.

First, let's talk about the physical signs. Digestive problems are one of the most common issues. If your vagus nerve isn't working right, you might have trouble going to the bathroom, feeling full, or eating. Why? For one main reason, the vagus nerve is important for gut motility, which are the wave-like muscle contractions that move food through your digestive system. Things can get backed up when it's not being used enough.

That's not all, though. Low vagal tone has also been linked to pain that can't be explained and feeling tired all the time. Are you always tired, even after a good night's sleep? Having aches and pains that you can't seem to pin down? These could be signs that your vagus nerve needs help.

For now, let's talk about feelings and thoughts. Have you been feeling more stressed out or sad lately? Are you finding it hard to focus or decide what to do? These could also be linked to a low vagus nerve tone. The vagus nerve is very closely linked to the parts of your brain that control your mood and your ability to think. It can leave you mentally and physically drained when it's not working at full speed.

More and more study is being done on the link between low vagal tone and mental health. A lot of the time, people who are depressed and anxious have lower vagal tone than people who don't have these illnesses. But it's clear that the vagus nerve has a big impact on our emotional health. More study is needed to fully understand this link.

Aside from the physical and mental, low vagal tone also has a social side to it. It can make it harder to connect with other people, understand how they feel, and keep our feelings in check when we're with other people. This is because the vagus nerve helps us understand and react to social cues accurately. Even if we don't mean to, we may come across as cold or uncaring when it's off.

So, don't give up if you're feeling any of these things. Getting your body's music back on track is easy and can be done in a number of ways. You can learn a lot of different techniques in the parts that follow, such as how to change your diet and do mindfulness meditation, as well as how to do   breathing   exercises.

Do not forget that this is not a quick fix. Rewiring your nervous system and getting your balance back takes time and regular work. But if you are patient and don't give up, you can help your body fix itself and get past the problems that   low   vagal   tone   can   cause.

How to Check How Well Your Vagus Nerve Works
Sometimes you might wonder if your vagus nerve is working right. You may have heard the phrase but not sure what it means for your health. So, get ready to go on a trip to find yourself! We'll show you how to test your vagus nerve function in this part, giving you the power to take charge of your health.

It's like an artery for communication—the vagus nerve links your brain and body in a lot of different ways. Everything about you is affected by it, from your mood and immune system to your heartbeat and nutrition. It's like having a director inside your head making sure that all the instruments play together nicely.

How can you tell if your conductor is at his or her best?
Here are some easy but useful self-tests that can help you figure out how healthy your vagus nerve is. A Test of Your Gag Reflex It may not seem exciting, but the gag response is a quick and easy way to check how well the vagus nerve is working. Open your mouth wide and touch the back of your throat softly with a toothbrush or cotton swab. It's a good sign if you want to gag. This means that your vagus nerve is working well.

The Variability Check of the Heart Rate The difference in time between your heartbeats is called heart rate variability (HRV). Your vagus nerve is a key part of a good HRV, which means your nervous system is in balance. You can track your HRV with apps or smart tech, or you can just count your pulse for 60 seconds and write down any changes. A steady beat that changes slightly over time is a good sign.

The Exercise for Being Aware of Breath Your vagus nerve is very close to your breath. Take a moment to focus on your breathing to figure out what it does. Pay attention to how deep and fast you breathe in and out. Does anything make you feel tense or limited? A deep, calm breath means that the vagus nerve is working well, while shallow or hurried breathing could mean that things could be better.

The Digestive Awareness Thoughts People often call their gut the "second brain," and it makes sense—the vagus nerve is a key part of digestion. Really pay attention to how you feel in your gut. Do you have trouble digesting food? Do you get gas, hurt, or have irregular bowel movements? A healthy vagus nerve is often linked to a happy gut.

The Check-In for Feelings The vagus nerve is very connected to how we feel. Think about how you're feeling right now. Is your mood stable and calm, or do you often feel anxious, stressed, or sad? A healthy vagus nerve and a balanced mental state often go hand in hand.

These are some easy ways to check how well your vagus nerve is working. Do not forget that evaluating yourself is only the beginning. If you see places where you could do better, don't give up! You can improve the operation of the vagus nerve in a number of ways, such as: Exercises for Deep Breathing: To calm your nervous system and awaken your vagus nerve, try box breathing, diaphragmatic breathing, or breathing through your alternate nostrils.

If you sing, hum, or chant, These things work the muscles in your throat and trigger the vagus nerve, which makes you feel calm and healthy. Yoga and meditation: Mind-body techniques like yoga and meditation can improve health by increasing the activity of the vagus nerve and lowering stress. Cold Exposure: Putting an ice pack on your neck or taking a cold shower can temporarily expose you to cold temperatures and make you stronger.

Social Connection: Laughing and having deep talks with loved ones can stimulate the vagus nerve and make you feel better.

Probiotics: These good bacteria help keep your gut healthy, which can then improve the function of your vagus nerve.

Remember that your body is always talking to you. You can learn a lot about the health of your vagus nerve by tuning in and listening to its messages. Now that you know this, you can make choices that will help this important nerve and allow your body to heal itself.

Why it's Important to Find Vagus Nerve Dysfunction
Your body's silent alarm

Think of your vagus nerve as a quiet alarm that keeps an eye on and controls the environment inside your body all the time. When everything works right, you don't even know it's there. Every instrument in a well-run orchestra plays its part in perfect rhythm, making a beautiful symphony of health and well-being. But when things start to go badly, this quiet alarm goes off to let you know something is wrong.

The Secret Killer

A dysfunctional vagus nerve is often the hidden cause of many long-term health issues, ranging from migraines and anxiety to sadness and digestive issues. A vagus nerve that isn't working right can cause a chain reaction of bad health effects all over the body, like a domino effect. A lot of people suffer for years without understanding that this important nerve is the cause of their problems.

Getting to Know the Bad Guy

Figuring out if your vagus nerve isn't working right is very important because it lets you fix the cause of your health problems instead of just the symptoms. You have to find the bad guy, the person who has been running things behind the scenes the whole time, like in a mystery story. Once you know who the bad guy is, you can take steps to make your body's internal environment balanced and harmonious again.

A Very Important Turning Point

Knowing the signs of a vagus nerve that isn't working right is a very important step in your healing process. It's like finding the last piece of the puzzle that was missing. It opens up a whole new world of options. Knowing how your vagus nerve works and how worry, trauma, and other things can affect it will give you the power to take charge of your health and well-being.

The Effect of Ripples

When the vagus nerve doesn't work right, it can affect many parts of the body, from your mood and energy to your gut and immune system. As if someone dropped a rock into a pond, it would make waves that went everywhere. If you can find and fix vagus nerve failure, you can stop these waves in their tracks and make your body's internal waters calm down again.

A Whole-Person Approach

It's good news that there are lots of things you can do to help your vagus nerve and get it functional again.

There is no quick fix. Instead, you need to take a more comprehensive approach that includes making changes to your lifestyle, dealing with stress, and doing things that help you relax and feel good. It's like taking care of a yard by feeding the soil, watering the plants, and making sure they have everything they need to grow.

Your body's ability to heal itself

Remember that your body can fix itself amazingly well. It is possible for your body to heal itself from the inside out if you can find out what is wrong with your vagus nerve and take steps to fix it. You're giving your body the tools it needs to fix and rebuild, which makes the base for your health and well-being stronger and more stable.

The Impact of the Butterfly

People often call the vagus nerve the "butterfly nerve" because it affects so many parts of the body. A butterfly moving its wings can change the weather all over the world. Similarly, a healthy vagus nerve can change your health and well-being for the better.

Getting your potential out

If you can find and fix vagus nerve dysfunction, you can help your body heal itself and make good changes in every part of your life. You can get rid of chronic pain, lower your stress and depression, and improve your health and well-being in general. It's like opening a door to a world of options.

Start your path to healing.

The process of getting your vagus nerve better might not be easy, but it is worth it. It's like going on a journey. You'll learn new things about your body and yourself, and you'll come back stronger and bigger than ever. Today, take the first step toward a healthier, happy you.

.

Chapter 4: Lifestyle Practices for Vagus Nerve Health

Breathing Techniques for Vagus Nerve Stimulation

As the saying goes, "breath is life." Did you know, though, that your breath could be your secret tool against mental health problems and long-term pain? For our first look into vagus nerve stimulation, let's do something easy but profound: breathe.

The vagus nerve, which is like a superhighway for your body's messages, is very important for controlling your stress reaction. This part of your brain sends calming signals when it is activated, which stops your fight-or-flight reaction. Now is the time when certain breathing methods really shine through.

How to Breathe Through Your Diaphragm: The Power of Deep Breaths

It's not just about filling your lungs when you do diaphragmatic breathing, which is also called belly breathing. You need to turn on your parasympathetic nervous system, which is your body's "rest and digest" mode. Picture this: you're on the ground with a book on your stomach. The book slowly rises when you breathe in and falls when you breathe out. This mental picture helps your diaphragm work, which is a dome-shaped muscle at the base of your lungs that is important for deep breathing.

Cortisol is your body's main stress hormone. Research has

shown that diaphragmatic breathing can lower it by a large amount. In a study that was released in the Journal of Alternative and Complementary Medicine, people who did diaphragmatic breathing for eight weeks felt less stressed and anxious. Imagine how powerful it would be to just take a few deep breaths.

Using alternate nostril breathing: Every breath is in tune As an important part of yogic techniques, alternate nostril breathing is known to help balance and calm the body. By switching the flow of air between your nose and mouth, you make a regular pattern that calms your nervous system.

Think of a gentle wave that goes up and down with each breath. By synchronizing the activity of both hemispheres of your brain, this rhythmic breathing can help you feel calm and aware.

It's not just about feeling good to do this. Studies have shown that breathing through the other nostril can improve your happiness, sharpen your mind, and even ease the pain of migraines and headaches. It's like a short meditation that you can do anywhere at any time. Making breathing exercises a part of your everyday life Do not undervalue the power of adding these breathing exercises to your daily practice.

It might be as easy as making time for five minutes of diaphragmatic breathing every morning or adding alternate nostril breathing to the things you do before bed. Always being the same is important. The more you do something, the easier it gets, just like any other skill. Imagine taking a few minutes to breathe deeply and mindfully to start your day. What do you think that will do for the rest of your day? Think about yourself relaxing in the evening by breathing through different nostrils. Could this routine take the place of that restless tossing and turning?

Do not believe what I say. Try it out and see for yourself how the power of breath can change things. Enjoy the process, be patient with yourself, and take pleasure in the trip. In the end, each breath is a gift, a chance to connect with your body and take care of your health.

Vagus Nerve Helper

We've looked at changes to our food, exercise, and the power of connection as ways to improve the health of our vagus nerve. Now, let's look inside your mind and see the beautiful scenery that is there. Mindfulness and meditation aren't just trendy words or ideas; they're powerful tools that can have a big effect on your vagus nerve and, by extension, your health.

Being aware of the present moment as medicine Imagine that you are sitting in a park with birds singing and the sun on your face. Are you fully in the present moment, or is your mind racing through a list of things to do, talks from the past, or worries about the future? Being mindful is the way to calm down this inner chaos. Being able to stay in the current moment and notice your feelings, thoughts, and sensations without judging them is an art.

What does this have to do with the vagus nerve?

Mindfulness techniques have been shown to raise vagal tone, which is a measure of how active the vagus nerve is. In turn, this has been linked to less stress, worry, and even swelling. Basically, when you're mindful, you tell your vagus nerve that everything is okay, which starts a chain of physiological reactions that make you feel better.

A Talk with Your Nervous System About Meditation
Mindfulness is about noticing things, and meditation is about becoming more aware of those things. One thing that you should always keep your mind on during meditation is one thing, like your breath, a phrase, or a picture in your mind. Even though it seems easy, this is a good way to work out your brain and make it less reactive and more adaptable.

For me, meditation is like having a straight line to my brain. Regular exercise can lower blood pressure, lower the stress hormone cortisol, and improve heart rate variability, which is another sign of a healthy vagus nerve. By massaging your vagus nerve from the inside out, you can picture what it feels like.

Helpful Hints to Get You Started

You don't have to be a monk or a yoga teacher to help yourself through meditation and awareness. Here are some easy ways to make these habits a part of your daily life:

• Begin Small: Daily meditation or focused breathing for just a few minutes can help. Find a quiet place, set a timer, and just watch your breath go in and out.
• Guided Meditations: There are a lot of apps and websites

that offer guided meditations. These can be very helpful for people who are just starting to meditate.

• Mindful Moments: Bring focus into the things you do every day. Enjoy every bite of food you eat. Pay attention to how your feet feel as you walk.
• Body Scan Meditation: To do this, slowly bring your attention to different parts of your body and notice any feelings without judging them. It helps you calm down and get in touch with your body.

As you practice loving-kindness meditation, you feel warm and compassionate toward yourself and others. It can help people feel connected and healthy.
• Be patient: To get better at awareness and meditation, you need to practice them. When your thought wanders, don't give up. Just bring your attention back to the present.

How inner peace can spread like a butterfly

Do not forget that your feelings and thoughts have a. Mindfulness and meditation aren't just good for relaxing your mind; they also help your vagus nerve and boost your body's natural ability to heal itself. For many, the ripple effects can be huge, causing less pain, better mood, and a stronger will to handle life's obstacles. Remember that your mind is a strong friend as you go on your journey. Not only will these habits change the way you think, but they will also change your life from the inside out.

Exercise and movement can help improve vagal tone.

Do you remember how calm and relaxed you felt after a great workout or a quick walk in the woods? You're not just making your muscles happy. It's also because your vagus nerve is singing a happy tune. Movement and exercise are great ways to improve vagal tone and get a lot of health benefits for your body and mind.

The Vagus Nerve Moves and Dances

Think of your vagus nerve as the director of the orchestra that is your body. Working out sets off a chain of events that affect everything from your mood and immune system to your heart rate and gut. It's like giving this important nerve a gentle massage, which makes it more flexible and sensitive.

Heart rate variability (HRV) is one of the most interesting ways that exercise changes the vagus nerve. The difference in time between heartbeats is measured by HRV. A higher HRV is usually linked to better vagal tone. Regular exercise has been shown to raise HRV, which means that the vagus nerve is stronger and more flexible.

But that's not the end of the good things. Endorphins are our body's natural painkillers and mood boosters. They are released when we exercise. The vagus nerve and these chemicals that make you feel good work together to lower worry, anxiety, and depression, giving you a sense of well-being and peace.

The best exercises for vagal tone can help you find your rhythm.

To improve vagal tone, there is no one-size-fits-all way to work out. The important thing is to find things you enjoy doing and can regularly fit into your schedule. However, it has been shown that some types of exercise are better than others at stimulating the vagus nerve. 1.Aerobic Exercise: You can get your heart rate up and your vagus nerve firing when you run, swim, ride a bike, or dance. Do moderate-intensity aerobic exercise for at least 30 minutes most days of the week to get the most out of it.

2.Mind-body practices like yoga and Tai Chi mix slow, gentle movements with deep breathing and awareness, making them ideal for improving vagal tone. Downward-facing dog and sun salutations are two yoga poses and Tai Chi moves that can help you relax by stimulating the vagus nerve.

3.Not only does strength training make you look good, it's also good for your vagus nerve. HRV and vagal tone can be improved by doing resistance activities like weightlifting and bodyweight training. This is especially true when combined with aerobic activity. 4.Doing things outside: Being in nature for a long time has a big effect on vagal tone. When you combine physical action with the healing power of nature, like when you hike, kayak, or garden, you get twice as many benefits.

Moving as Medicine: More Than Just the Gym

Movement is a great way to improve vagal tone, and you don't have to go to the gym or follow a set exercise plan. A big change can be made by just adding more movement to your daily life.

Stick to the stairs instead of the lift.

• Park farther away from where you want to go and walk the rest of the way.

• Move around your living room while listening to your favorite music.

• Stretch while you're at work.

• Have fun with your kids or pets.

Moving around in small ways makes you healthier and happy in the long run.

What Exercise Does to Your Body

You're not just building your muscles and improving your heart health when you make exercise and movement a priority. In addition, you're giving your vagus nerve a much-needed boost, which has good effects all over your body and mind.

Better vagal tone can help you sleep better, lower inflammation, digest food better, and even make your immune system stronger. The feeling of well-being and energy spreads through your whole body like a wave. Put on your shoes, roll out your yoga mat, or just go for a walk outside. Let your vagus nerve lead you to the best health and happiness possible, and use exercise as medicine.

What Sleep and Relaxation Do for You

You've probably heard the saying "rest and digest," but have you ever thought about what it means for the health of your vagus nerve? Relaxing and getting enough sleep are not just nice to have; they are important parts of a healthy living that can have a big effect on how well your vagus nerve works.

Sleep is the body's natural way to start over. Sleep is like having a repair crew come in at night to fix things. Your brain is busy getting rid of waste, fixing cells, and putting memories together while you sleep. That's not all, though. Sleep is also very important for keeping your stress reaction in check.

The stress hormone cortisol is made more by your body when you don't get enough sleep. When your cortisol levels are too high, they can mess up your vagus nerve, making it less able to control your body's processes.

Good sleep, on the other hand, lowers cortisol levels and raises melatonin levels, which is a hormone that helps you relax and sleep. For the vagus nerve to work well, this chemical balance is very important. How sleep works and what the vagus nerve does A strong link has been found between the quality of sleep and the function of the vagus nerve.

Researchers have found that people who have problems sleeping, like sleeplessness, often have less activity in their vagus nerve than people who sleep well. Getting better sleep has also been shown to make the vagus nerve work more. This suggests that putting sleep first can be a great way to improve the function of your vagus nerve and enjoy all of its benefits.

How to Relax and Feel Better

Another important part of the vagus nerve game is that you need to relax. The "fight or flight" reaction is set off by your sympathetic nervous system when you're busy or stressed. This reaction is meant to help you deal with immediate threats, but if it happens all the time, it can hurt your vagus nerve.

Deep breathing, yoga, and other forms of relaxation can help to engage your parasympathetic nervous system. This is the "rest and digest" part of your nervous system that works with your sympathetic nervous system. This activity tells your vagus nerve to calm down, which lowers stress and improves your health as a whole.

Other Lifestyle Factors Besides Sleep and Relaxation

Sleep and rest are important for the health of the vagus nerve, but other things in your life can also affect it. Better vagus nerve activity has been linked to regular exercise, a healthy diet high in omega-3 fatty acids, and spending time with friends and family.

Tips for Better Sleep and Relaxation: How to Use Them
• Make a regular sleep routine. Every day, even on the weekends, go to bed and wake up at the same time. For example, don't look at a computer for at least an hour before bed. Instead, take a warm bath or read a book.
• Make sure your bedroom is cool, dark, and quiet so you can sleep well.

• Put calming techniques at the top of your list: do yoga, deep breathing exercises, or meditation every day.
• Get to know other people: spend time with family and friends, join a social group, or do volunteer work.

The Effects of Rest on Chains

Remember that your vagus nerve is like a butterfly's wings—it can send waves through your body. Putting sleep and rest first will not only help your vagus nerve work better, but it will also start a chain of good changes that will improve your health and well-being as a whole.

Imagine waking up feeling calm and peaceful inside, like you've been given new life. Imagine being able to handle the tasks in life with more strength and ease. This is what a healthy vagus nerve can do, and you can get it.

Take the time to learn how to rest and relax. It should be an important part of your daily life. Your body and mind will feel better, and your vagus nerve will thank you.

What you eat and the vagus nerve: feeding your "butterfly"

People often say, "You are what you eat," but have you ever thought about how this really affects your vagus nerve? Our body's internal "butterfly," this strong nerve, is closely linked to our gut system and is greatly affected by the foods we eat. In the same way that a butterfly needs the right food to grow, your vagus nerve needs certain nutrients to be in good health.

A Symphony of Tastes for Healthy Vagus Nerves

Think of your diet as a symphony, with each food group playing a different part. A beautiful song is made when all the instruments work together. In this case, a healthy vagus nerve and a body buzzing with happiness. Let us look at the main players in this nutritional orchestra:

• "The Omega-3 Overture": Flaxseeds, walnuts, fatty fish (salmon, mackerel, sardines), and other foods high in omega-3 fatty acids are great for reducing inflammation. According to research, they may increase the activity of the vagus nerve, which may help keep your mood stable, lower your nervousness, and even ease the pain of migraines. You can think of them as the violins in our orchestra that set a calm tone.

• The Prebiotic and Probiotic Duet: Prebiotics, which are found in foods like garlic, onions, and bananas, and probiotics, which are found in foods like yogurt, kefir, and sauerkraut, both help the gut microbiome, which is the group of microorganisms that live in our digestive tract. The vagus nerve and a healthy microbiome talk to each other, which helps the gut-brain connection work well. These people play the woodwinds in our symphony and give it more depth and variety.

• The Zinc Solo: Zinc is a nutrient that is found in meat, shellfish, beans, and nuts. It is very important for the vagus nerve to send messages. It has been linked that getting enough zinc can lower inflammation and help your happiness. Think of it as the trumpet, which plays clear, resonant sounds.

• The B Vitamin Ensemble: B vitamins, especially B12 (found in meat, fish, and eggs), are important for nerve health, and the vagus nerve is one of them. They help the body make neurotransmitters, use energy, and stay healthy in general. They keep the rhythm strong and steady, so think of them as the percussion part.

• The Polyphenol Chorus: Green tea, berries, and many colorful fruits and veggies are full of polyphenols, which are powerful antioxidants that keep the vagus nerve from getting hurt. They add richness and life to our music like a choir.

Be careful with these foods: they can upset the balance. Some foods can throw off the vagus nerve in the same way that an out of tune note can ruin a song. Too much caffeine, highly processed foods, and refined sugars can all cause inflammation and mess up the gut bacteria, which makes the vagus nerve less effective. It's best to eat whole, raw foods as much as possible and in moderation.

Feeding your "butterfly" for the best health Remember that the food you eat isn't just to satisfy your hunger; it's to fuel your whole body. By giving your vagus nerve the right nutrients, you not only help it work at its best, but you also boost your body's natural ability to heal itself.

Enjoy the variety of tastes that nature offers, try out new recipes, and enjoy the pleasure of feeding your "butterfly." Doing so will unleash a chain of positive effects, from better sleep and less stress to higher resilience and happier moods. It's truly on your plate what you can do to change your health.

Chapter 5: Vagus Nerve Stimulation Techniques: Singing, Humming, Chanting, and Gargling

Get ready to release your inner bird of song and find healing music! We're going to talk about the magical link between your voice, your vagus nerve, and your health in general in this section. If you sing in the shower or hum in the bathroom, you're about to be amazed at how simple sounds can positively affect your health.

The sound you make is a vagus nerve VIP

What did you know about the vagus nerve? It goes straight to your vocal cords and the muscles at the back of your throat. It's like getting a backstage pass to the most exclusive performance for your nervous system! You're basically giving your vagus nerve a gentle push when you sing, hum, chant, or even gargle. This activates those muscles and sets off a chain of good things that happen all over your body.

How Sound Can Help Your Health

Scientists have found that these vocal sounds can make your heart rate variability (HRV) higher. HRV is a way to measure how flexible and strong your nervous system is. If your HRV is high, your body is better able to deal with stress and get back on its feet after problems. Also, guess what? It has been shown that singing, humming, and chanting raise HRV and vagal tone. This is a fancy way of saying that your vagus nerve is working at full capacity.

Sing your way to peace.

You have to harmonize your mind, body, and spirit when you sing. It's not enough to just hit the right notes. Endorphins and oxytocin are two hormones in your brain that make you feel good. When you sing, they flood your body. You can get rid of stress, anxiety, and sadness with these natural mood boosters. They will make you feel good and give you energy. Anytime you sing, whether it's your favorite pop song or with a choir, it's a strong way to connect with your feelings and be creative.

A good habit is humming.

It's great to hum if you're not quite ready for a single performance. It stimulates the vagus nerve in your voice. When you hum, a soft vibration happens in your throat and head that can help you rest and calm down. It feels a lot like getting a massage for your vagus nerve! You could hum a simple song while you do the dishes, go for a walk, or just sit back and relax. It will surprise you how quickly this easy exercise can calm your mind and make your body feel better.

Chanting: Using Ancient Wisdom to Improve Your Health Today

For hundreds of years, people have used chanting as a spiritual and mental tool to help them feel better and find inner peace. Chanting's repeated beats and sounds can put you in a trance-like state, which can calm your mind and turn on your parasympathetic nervous system, which is the "rest and digest" part of your nervous system. Chanting, whether you use a traditional mantra or just say a positive statement over and over, can be a very effective way to relieve stress, improve focus, and find inner peace.

A Surprising Way to Hack the Vagus Nerve

You read that right! Not only does gargling help sore throats, it's also a surprisingly good way to activate your vagus nerve. When you gargle, you work out the muscles in the back of your throat. These muscles send messages along the vagus nerve, which can help calm your nervous system and reduce swelling. If you're worried or sick, grab that mouthwash and gargle your vagus nerve!

Adding Vocal Vagus Nerve Stimulation to Your Everyday Life

These methods are great because they are easy to use, fun, and accessible. You only need your voice and a desire to try new things. No training or special tools are needed. If you want to add vocal vagus nerve stimulation to your everyday life, here are some ideas: Start your day with a song. You can sing in the shower, hum along to the radio, or chant a statement to make the day start off on a good note.

• Take a break to hum. If you're worried or overwhelmed, hum a soothing song for a few minutes.
• Join a singing group: Singing in a band or group can help you meet new people and improve your health.

• Make gargling a daily habit. To give your vagus nerve a

daily boost, gargle with warm salt water or mouthwash after you brush your teeth.

• Try singing: Try out different ways of chanting to find one that feels right to you.

Remember that the most important thing is to do what works for you every day. You'll be amazed at how these easy sounds can change your health and happiness if you practice them and wait.

Being exposed to cold (like cold showers or ice packs)
When you expose yourself to cold, it plays a surprisingly powerful role in your body's natural healing process. It might not make sense—aren't we designed to look for warmth and comfort? But if you are exposed to cold in small amounts, it can make a big difference, especially when it comes to activating and training your vagus nerve.

People who are interested in health and fitness have probably told you about cold showers or ice baths. These habits aren't just short-lived trends; they have deep roots in ancient cultures and are now backed by more and more scientific proof. The idea behind it is simple: when your body feels cold, it responds in ways that set off your vagus nerve, which sets off a chain of positive physiological responses.

Think about getting a cold shower. At first, it might be a shock, but as you get used to it, your heart rate slows, your breath gets deeper, and you feel calm. That's the vagus nerve at work. It's telling your body that it's time to unwind, calm down, and recover.

According to research, being in the cold can make the vagus nerve work a lot more. So, this can slow down the fight-or-flight reaction, lower inflammation, and make you feel better all around. You can step back from the chaos of daily life and connect with your body's natural knowledge. It's like pressing the "reset" button on your nervous system.

But that's not the end of the good things. Being outside in the cold has also been linked to better blood flow, a stronger immune system, and even a faster metabolism. You can easily get this tool, but it can have huge effects on your mental and physical health. Right now, before you rush to take an ice bath, let's look at some easy and useful ways to expose yourself to cold every day.

A refreshing way to start the day is with a cold shower. A cold shower is a great way to start if you're not used to being cold. It's a gentle way to get your body used to how cold can make you feel better. Start lowering the warmth of your shower slowly as you get to the end. Over time, you can stay in the cold water for longer periods of time. Remember that the goal is not to survive the coldest level, but to find a level that feels hard but doable.

Ice packs are a targeted way to ease pain and swelling. Ice packs can be used to protect a specific area from the cold. You can put them on certain parts of your body to ease pain and swelling. For instance, putting an ice pack on your face or neck can help ease the pain of a migraine.

Putting your body in cold water: a deeper look at vagus nerve stimulation

Cold water immersion is a great choice for people who want a more intense experience. You can do this by swimming in a cold lake or ocean, taking an ice bath, or even putting your face in a bowl of ice water. Immersion in cold water can make the vagus nerve reaction stronger, which can help you relax more deeply and feel less stressed.

When starting a new habit, it's important to pay attention to your body and move slowly. Start by being exposed to the cold for short amounts of time and slowly lengthen the time as your body gets used to it. Before starting a cold exposure practice, you should always talk to your doctor if you already have any health problems.

Adding exposure to cold into your daily life can change you in big ways. It's a way to get in touch with your body's natural healing powers, feel less stressed, and improve your overall health. At first, it might be a little cold, but the benefits are worth it. When you accept the power of cold, you'll feel stronger and more alive, both physically and mentally.

Acupuncture and acupressure to stimulate the vagus nerve

Are you interested in the ancient arts of acupuncture and massage and how they might help you get the most out of your vagus nerve? These tried-and-true methods, which

come from traditional Chinese medicine, are a unique and effective way to trigger the vagus nerve and use its amazing healing   powers.
Acupuncture is an old way to heal.

For acupuncture to work, thin needles are carefully put into certain spots on the body, which are called acupoints. Meridians, which are thought to be paths of energy flow, run through these acupoints. Researchers are still trying to figure out how acupuncture works, but they think it might stimulate the vagus nerve and set off a chain of positive effects.

One amazing thing about acupuncture is that it can change the way the nerve system works. The autonomic nervous system, which is led by the vagus nerve, can be stimulated by acupuncture by focusing on certain acupoints. When this action happens, it can make you feel calmer, less stressed, and better overall. Acupuncture is like a gentle push that tells your vagus nerve to take charge and lead your body to balance   and   unity.
A lot of research has shown that acupuncture may be able to stimulate the vagus nerve. For instance, studies have shown that acupuncture can raise vagal tone, which is a measure of how active the vagus nerve is, in people with different health problems. This rise in vagal tone has been linked to less inflammation, better heart rate fluctuations, and better control of emotions.

Acupressure: Use your fingertips to heal

Not to worry if the thought of needles makes you a little queasy! Acupressure is a way to trigger the vagus nerve that doesn't involve needles. You can use the same mending processes as acupuncture by gently pressing on certain acupoints. You can take care of your vagus nerve health with acupressure, which is like do-it-yourself acupuncture.

Acupressure, like acupuncture, can help you rest, lower your stress, and feel better all around. With this easy but effective tool, you can make it a part of your daily life. If you need a moment of peace and quiet or are feeling stressed or overwhelmed, acupressure can help. It's a gentle way to connect with your body's natural healing knowledge.

Acupoints to stimulate the vagus nerve

Different acupoints on the body can be treated with acupuncture and acupressure, but some points work especially well for stimulating the vagus nerve. Some of these are:

• Stomach 36 (ST36): This acupoint is important for your health and well-being and is located below the kneecap. Stimulating ST36 can raise vagal tone, lower inflammation, and give you more energy.

• Pericardium 6 (PC6): This part of the body is on the inside of the wrist and is known to calm and ease nausea. The vagus nerve can be stimulated, which can help you relax.

• Large Intestine 4 (LI4): This acupoint is on the hand and is used for many things, such as relieving pain and boosting the immune system. The tone of the vagus nerve can also be improved by stimulating LI4.

•Ear Shen Men: This acupoint is called "Divine Gate" in Chinese. It's at the very top of the triangular fossa in the ear and is known for its ability to calm and ease pain. This acupoint may be stimulated to improve the flow of "Qi," or life force energy, to the brain. This may help the vagus nerve become active.

How Acupuncture and Acupressure Work Together
As you start your acupuncture and acupressure path, keep in mind that even small changes can have a big impact on your health. Every time you stimulate your vagus nerve, you not only make yourself feel better and more relaxed right now, but you also set yourself up for a healthier, happy future.

If you choose acupuncture, acupressure, or a mix of the two, these old techniques can help your body heal itself quite effectively. So why not give them a shot? Once the vagus nerve is activated, it will have the butterfly effect and change your life one gentle touch at a time.

Massage and other bodywork therapies can help your vagus nerve feel better.

We've tried a lot of different methods, from breathwork to food changes, to find out how to heal the vagus nerve. Now let's explore the world of touch treatment. Massage and bodywork can send a message deep into your vagus nerve that makes you feel calm and at ease. Touch is more than just touching.

Touch is a basic language that lets us talk to each other without words. To soothe, heal, and connect us to our bodies and feelings, touch is powerful. It can be the soft touch of a loved one or the firm pressure of a massage therapist's hands.

Massage and other bodywork therapies have been shown to have a good effect on the vagus nerve, making it stronger and helping people feel calm and relaxed. Some pressure points and nerve endings are stimulated in these treatments. This sends signals to the brain that turn on the parasympathetic nervous system, which is part of the autonomic nervous system and is known as the "rest and digest" system.
Different kinds of massage and bodywork that stimulate the vagus nerve

Here are some well-known massage and bodywork techniques that are known to trigger the vagus nerve:
• Swedish Massage: Long, flowing strokes, kneading, and friction are used in this traditional massage style to ease muscle tension, improve circulation, and lower stress.

• Deep Tissue Massage: This type of therapeutic massage works on the deeper layers of muscle and connective tissue to relieve tension and help you rest.

• Myofascial Release: This method is all about loosening

up the fascia, which is the connective tissue that covers muscles and glands.

• Craniosacral treatment: This gentle, hands-on treatment works with the rhythms of the skull, spine, and cerebrospinal fluid, which make up the craniosacral system.

• Reflexology: In this treatment, pressure is put on certain points on the feet or hands that are thought to represent different body systems and organs.

• Acupressure: In this form of traditional Chinese medicine, you press on certain places along energy meridians to help your body heal and stay balanced.

How massage and other bodywork therapies can help the vagus nerve

Massage and other bodywork treatments can help stimulate the vagus nerve in many different ways. It has been shown that these treatments can Massage has been shown to lower cortisol levels, which is the "stress hormone," and raise serotonin and dopamine levels, which are the "feel-good" chemicals.

• Get rid of pain: Massage can help get rid of pain by increasing blood flow, calming muscles, and making the body release endorphins, which are natural painkillers.
• Help you sleep better: Massage can help you relax and sleep better by lowering your stress, worry, and pain.
• Make your immune system stronger: massage can make

natural killer cells work harder. These are a type of white blood cell that is very important for the immune system.

As a result of massage, the parasympathetic nervous system can be activated. This increases blood flow to the digestive organs and encourages peristalsis, the wave-like muscle contractions that move food through the digestive track.

How to Pick the Best Massage or Bodywork Therapy for You

With all the different kinds of massage and bodywork treatments out there, it's important to pick one that fits your needs. When making your choice, think about your own preferences, health, and finances.

Talk to a trained massage therapist or bodywork practitioner if you don't know where to begin. These people can help you figure out which therapy will work best for your wants and goals.

Adding massage and other bodywork techniques to your routine for vagus nerve stimulation

Adding massage and other bodywork therapies to your schedule for stimulating the vagus nerve can be very helpful. Incorporating touch therapy into your everyday life can have a huge effect on your health, whether you get a massage from a professional or do it yourself at home. Always being the same is important. Try to get a massage or other treatment done regularly, whether that's once a week, once a month, or more often if that works better for you. To further stimulate your vagus nerve and help you relax throughout the day, you can also do self-massages like stroking, squeezing, or tapping to go along with professional massages.

As you start this journey of touch and healing, keep in mind that your body is a temple and that massage and other bodywork treatments are sacred ceremonies that honor its strength and wisdom. By using touch to care for your vagus nerve, you open up a source of self-healing power that can lead to a life full of health, happiness, and energy.

Yoga and Tai Chi for Stimulating the Vagus Nerve: A Healing Symphony for the Mind and Body

We will learn about the old practices of yoga and tai chi in this chapter. These are two gentle but effective ways to help strengthen and stimulate the vagus nerve. These tried-and-true practices combine movement, breath, and awareness in a way that works well together. This creates a symphony of healing waves that reach deep into our nervous system.

Asana: A Calm Dance with the Vagus Nerve

With all of its different styles and forms, yoga has a huge number of poses (asanas) and breathing routines (pranayama) that can have a direct effect on the vagus nerve. As we do these poses, we not only stretch and strengthen our bodies, but we also rub our organs, which stimulates the vagus nerve fibers that run through them.

Let's look at some specific yoga poses that have been shown to make the vagus nerve work better:

• Alternate Nostril Breathing (Nadi Shodhana Pranayama): This simple but profound practice involves breathing through each nostril alternatively. This helps to balance the nervous system and makes you feel calm and relaxed. Researchers have found that Nadi Shodhana can raise vagus tone, which is a key sign of a healthy vagus nerve.

• Lion's Breath (Simhasana Pranayama): To do this fun but strong exercise, stick out your tongue and roar like a lion. It may sound silly, but it's actually good for your vagus nerve. Lion's breath works the muscles in the throat and neck by forcing air out very quickly. This stimulates the vagus nerve and helps you relax.

Chanting (OM or AUM): When chanted with purpose, the ancient sound of OM can make vibrations that connect with the vagus nerve and make you feel calm and healthy. Research has shown that singing can lower stress hormones and raise vagal tone.

• Restorative yoga poses: Child's Pose, Legs-up-the-Wall Pose, and Reclining Bound Angle Pose are all supported, gentle poses that help you relax deeply. This lets the parasympathetic nervous system, which is led by the vagus nerve, take over and bring the body and mind back into balance.

• Sun Salutations (Surya Namaskar): This lively set of poses can wake up the vagus nerve, which can improve circulation and make the digestive system work better if done slowly and with awareness.

Remember to listen to your body and respect its knowledge as you start your yoga journey. Pick practices that feel good to you and change them as needed to fit your needs and skills.

Moving in a meditative way is Tai Chi.

Tai chi is a graceful martial art that mixes deep breathing, slow, flowing movements, and being aware of the present moment. It is often called "meditation in motion." This gentle practice has been shown to improve balance, lower stress, and boost the immune system, among other health benefits.

Tai chi's slow, deliberate movements trigger the vagus nerve, which makes you feel calm and less anxious. Tai chi includes deep breathing movements that make the vagus nerve work better. This raises the tone of the vagus nerve and makes you feel calm.

Researchers have found that tai chi can improve HRV, which is a key sign of how healthy the vagus nerve is. The difference in time between heartbeats is called HRV. A higher HRV means that your nervous system is healthy and more resilient.

Besides being good for your body, tai chi can also help your mind and spirit, which can improve the function of your vagus nerve. By doing tai chi, you learn to let go of worries and other things that aren't important in the present time. This practice of awareness can help calm the mind and the body, which can lead to relaxation and health.

The Link to the Vagus Nerve

Yoga and tai chi both work on the vagus nerve in a broad way, stimulating it on many levels to make it work better. The breathing and movement exercises directly stimulate the vagus nerve. The awareness and relaxation parts of these practices make it work even better.

Adding yoga and tai chi to your daily life can help strengthen your vagus nerve and let your body heal itself. Building a stronger bond between your mind and body will give you a fresh sense of peace, strength, and harmony.

So, get out your yoga mat or join the peaceful flow of tai chi. Welcome these practices' gentle power and let them lead you on a path of healing and change. You will be able to feel more joy, resilience, and good health as you improve your vagus nerve.

Chapter 6: Vagus Nerve Therapies and Interventions

Biofeedback for Vagus Nerve Training

We come across a lot of different tools and methods as we try to use the vagus nerve's power. Out of these, biofeedback stands out as an interesting and useful method. Biofeedback for training the vagus nerve is like looking in a mirror to see how we're feeling on the inside. It tells us about our body's processes in real time. This knowledge gives us the power to consciously change things we thought were out of our hands before.

What does biofeedback mean? As its basic form, biofeedback is a mind-body method that uses electronic devices to track and show body functions like heart rate, muscle tension, skin temperature, and even brainwave activity. After this, we are shown or told this information, which lets us see or hear how our thoughts, feelings, and actions affect the way our bodies work. We learn a lot about how our mind and body are connected through this feedback loop, and we learn how to make small changes that will improve our general health.

Biofeedback for Vagus Nerve Training: When biofeedback is used for vagus nerve training, it focuses on certain physiological signs that are linked to vagus nerve activity, like heart rate variability (HRV). HRV is the change in the amount of time that passes between heartbeats. A higher HRV means that you can better control your emotions and bounce back from setbacks. On the other hand, a lower

HRV is often linked to stress, worry, and long-term health problems.

We can learn to raise our HRV with biofeedback. This makes the vagus nerve stronger and turns on the parasympathetic nervous system. This can cause a chain reaction of good things to happen, such as less stress, better happiness, stronger immune system, and even less chronic pain.

How does it work? In order to train the vagus nerve through biofeedback, monitors are usually put on the body to track heart rate and other physiological factors. The data from these sensors is sent to a computer or other device that shows it right away. Your HRV may be shown on a graph, a tone may change pitch based on your HRV, or you may even be able to play a game that is driven by your body. Together with the help of a trained therapist, you learn to spot trends in your body's responses and try out various methods to change your HRV. Some of these methods are mindfulness meditation, guided imagery, deep breathing exercises, and even just noticing how your body reacts without judging it.

Biofeedback for vagus nerve training is like any other skill: you need to practice it a lot to get good at it. If you practice this method regularly, you will get better at picking up on subtle cues from your body and making changes to improve your health. You can teach your body to handle worry better over time, improve your emotional control, and develop a greater sense of calm and well-being.

Real-World Uses: Biofeedback is useful for training the vagus nerve in many places besides the treatment room. This method has been shown to help with many different health problems, such as anxiety, sadness, chronic pain, migraines, irritable bowel syndrome (IBS), and even post-traumatic stress disorder (PTSD).

For instance, research has shown that biofeedback can help people with anxiety learn to control their breathing and heart rate, which can make their anxiety feelings better. In the same way, biofeedback has been shown to help people with depression feel better and less depressed.

Beyond the Basics: Variability in heart rate is the main focus of biofeedback for training the vagus nerve, but other physiological factors may also be worked on. Some types of biofeedback may focus on things like skin temperature, muscle tightness, or even brainwave activity. These methods can help you understand your body's state better and give you new ways to control your own behavior.

What's Next for Biofeedback? As technology keeps getting better, biofeedback's uses are quickly growing. Biofeedback is getting easier to use, more interesting, and more successful by adding new sensors, algorithms, and interfaces. For example, more and more people are using wearable devices that track changes in heart rate and give real-time input. You can keep an eye on your body's state all day with these gadgets and practice self-regulation skills whenever and wherever you want.

Accept the trip: Using biofeedback to train your vagus nerve is like going on a trip to learn more about yourself and gain power. It's possible to heal, grow, and change in many ways once you learn to pay attention to your body's cues and use the power of your mind. Don't forget that the way you get there is just as important as the end goal. Accept that things will take time, be kind to yourself, and enjoy each small win along the way.

Transcutaneous Vagus Nerve Stimulation (tVNS): A Soft Buzz and a Strong Wizz

Transcutaneous vagus nerve stimulation (tVNS) could be your new best friend if you want to help your vagus nerve without hurting it. The gadget could be small enough to fit in your pocket and could send mild electrical signals through your skin to massage the vagus nerve. It's not science fiction; this is the real, exciting world of tVNS.

There are many signals that make up tVNS.

VNS is beautiful because it is so easy to use. The most common type of tVNS affects the auricular branch of the vagus nerve, which is found in your ear. A small gadget that looks like an earbud clips onto your ear and sends out mild electrical pulses. People say that these pulses feel like a small tingling or buzzing. They are not painful.

But don't be fooled by how gentle they are. These tiny messages are strong enough to turn on the vagus nerve, which then causes a chain of good things to happen in your body. Like dropping a pebble into a pond—a small move

that   makes   a   big   difference.
More Than Just a Tingle: What tVNS Could Do

The study of tVNS is still going on and is growing very quickly, but the results we have seen so far are very interesting. tVNS has shown promise in treating a number of diseases, such as :

Brain Pain and Migraines: Several studies show that tVNS may help lower the number and severity of migraines, which could help people who suffer from these painful headaches.

Depression and anxiety: tVNS has been shown to help some people with depression and anxiety issues, so it could be used to help people with these common mental health problems.

Pain that doesn't go away: Studies show that tVNS may help ease chronic pain, especially neuropathic pain (pain caused by nerve damage).

seizures: More research is needed, but some studies show that tVNS might be a useful extra treatment for people who have seizures.

The Benefits of tVNS: Giving You Power on Your Health   Journey
One of the best things about tVNS is how easy it is to get to and use. You can use tVNS in your daily life because the

gadgets are small and easy to use. You don't have to go to the clinic or see a doctor to trigger your vagus nerve.

You can do it while reading a book, working at your desk, or even just sitting on the couch.

tVNS is also usually thought to be safe and well-tolerated, and there have been few reports of side effects. Some people may have mild skin irritation or a short-term change in their hearing, but these are generally only minor side effects that go away on their own.

tVNS: A Supplement for Your Health

Keep in mind that tVNS is not a miracle cure or an alternative to regular medical care. However, it can be a useful addition to your health toolbox and give you the power to be involved in your own health journey. Ask your doctor or another health care provider about tVNS to find out if it's right for you.

Remember that your body is amazingly strong and able to heal itself. When you try treatments like tVNS, you're not just treating your symptoms; you're also boosting your body's natural ability to heal itself. A soft touch and a deep impact:

tVNS shows how powerful gentle actions can be. We can stimulate the vagus nerve and start a chain of good things happening in the body and mind by using the gentle power of electricity. Feel the tingle and the soft buzz that comes from tVNS. It will lead you to better health.

Vagus Nerve Implants (for Really Bad Cases)

Your body's main communication highway, the vagus nerve, is very important for controlling your mood, pain, and general health. Non-invasive therapies and changes to a person's lifestyle often have good effects, but sometimes a stronger intervention is needed.

Vagus nerve implants have become a beacon of hope for people with severe conditions that don't respond to treatment. They give them a way to recover their lives from the grips of their crippling symptoms.

How Vagus Nerve Implants Work

A vagus nerve implant, also called a vagus nerve stimulator (VNS), is a small, battery-powered device that is physically put under the chest skin. It works a lot like a pacemaker. From the machine to the vagus nerve in the neck is a thin line. The implant sends out small electrical pulses that stimulate the nerve. These pulses change the nerve's signals, which has a good effect all over the body.

When Should Vagus Nerve Implants Be Thought About?

Vagus nerve implants are usually only given to people with serious conditions that haven't improved with other treatments. Among these are:

Treatment-Resistant Epilepsy: VNS has been shown to greatly lower the number of seizures in people with epilepsy who don't react to medication. Treatment-Resistant Depression: VNS can make a huge difference in the lives of people with major depressive disorder who haven't gotten better with traditional treatments.

Other Conditions: VNS is also being studied for its possible benefits in a number of other conditions, such as chronic pain, headaches, inflammatory bowel disease, and post-traumatic stress disorder (PTSD). How implants for the vagus nerve do their magic Researchers are still trying to figure out exactly how VNS works to help people, but they have found a few key pathways:

Neurotransmitter Modulation: VNS is thought to make more neurotransmitters, such as serotonin and norepinephrine, which are very important for controlling mood.

Anti-Inflammatory Effects: The immune system and the vagus nerve are closely linked. VNS has been shown to lower inflammation all over the body, which may be one reason why it helps with many conditions. Brain Plasticity: VNS may help the brain make new neural connections and pathways, which makes it more resilient and able to adjust.

How Vagus Nerve Implants Can Change Things

Vagus nerve implants are not a miracle cure, but they could make a huge difference in the quality of life for people with serious diseases that don't respond to treatment. Imagine a life where your crippling seizures happen less often and aren't as bad, where your sadness isn't so heavy, and where your chronic pain doesn't control everything you do. Implants in the vagus nerve can make these dreams come true.

A Story of Hope and Comfort

Look at the story of Sarah, a woman who had serious epilepsy and had been sick for years. Even though she tried many medicines, her seizures were still out of control, which made her feel alone and helpless. Sarah went through an amazing change after having a VNS implanted. Her seizures got less regular and not as bad, and she was finally able to get her life back. Sarah's story is not the only one like it. Vagus nerve devices have helped a huge number of people feel better and give them new hope. The road to healing might not always be smooth, but the benefits could be huge.

Looking forward to a better future

If you or someone you care about has a serious illness that other treatments haven't helped, don't give up. Implants that connect to the vagus nerve could lead to a better future. Check with your doctor to see if VNS is a good choice for you. Don't forget that you're not on this trip by yourself. You can get through even the hardest problems and get your life back with the right help and treatment.

Another new treatment is whispering to the vagus nerve through the ear.

We have found a wealth of both well-known and new techniques that can be used to treat health problems by exploring the vagus nerve. We have talked about the power of breathwork, the relaxing embrace of yoga, and the dance-like flow of exercise. But that's not the end of our trip. Therapies for the vagus nerve are always changing as new methods are studied and found to work better. An exciting way to do this is to stimulate the vagus nerve through the ear.

The link between the ear and vagus nerve: a direct path to health

The ear has a surprising secret that isn't often talked about when people talk about health and healing. It's home to a branch of the vagus nerve, which gives you direct access to this powerful network of nerves. New treatments are using this link to their advantage by stimulating the ear gently to change the activity of the vagus nerve. This new way of doing things seems like it could help with a lot of different problems, from migraines and nervousness to chronic pain and inflammation.

TAVNS stands for transcutaneous auricular vagus nerve stimulation. It is a gentle touch.

The transcutaneous auricular vagus nerve stimulation (taVNS) method looks like one of the best options. Using this non-invasive method, small electrodes are placed on certain parts of the ear to trigger the vagus nerve with mild electrical impulses. According to research, taVNS may affect many bodily processes, such as the release of neurotransmitters like dopamine and serotonin and the rate at which the heart beats. The great thing about taVNS is how easy it is to use. Unlike implantable devices, taVNS can be given at home using portable devices, which gives people more control over their mending process. taVNS has been studied as a possible way to help people with migraines, anxiety, sadness, and even post-traumatic stress disorder (PTSD).

Imagine a world where a simple device you could keep in your home could help you deal with long-term pain, anxiety, or sadness. These are the things that taVNS could do. In this world, you can talk to your vagus nerve through your ear and gently push it toward balance and health.

The Future of Ear-Based Vagus Nerve Therapies After taVNS
While taVNS is the most popular, it's not the only ear-based vagus nerve therapy that's coming out soon. Acoustic vibrations and even light massage of certain ear points are other types of stimulation that researchers are looking into. It's still early days for these techniques, but they give us a taste of the exciting things that are to come.

Imagine a world where your vagus nerve could be used to fix you with a soothing melody, a gentle vibration, or a simple massage. This is the goal that drives people who work in and study this area. This is a picture of a world where the ear is a way to get to a healthy, happier, and more vibrant you.

How to Find Your Way to Vagus Nerve Healing with the Power of Choice

Therapies for the vagus nerve are very different and are always growing. There are many choices, from yoga and breathwork to exercise and ear-based stimulation. The choices are as different as the people who want them. There isn't a single method that works for everyone. The important thing is to look around, try different things, and see what works for you. Don't forget that your path to health is unique. It means paying attention to your body, meeting its needs, and getting the tools you need to take care of your health and well-being. You can choose between the gentle touch of taVNS, the steady flow of breathwork, or the cozy hug of yoga.

Remember that you are not alone as you start this journey. There are more and more people like you who are using the vagus nerve to create positive changes in their lives. Let's change the story of health and healing one breath, one movement, and one gentle touch at a time.

Chapter 7: Overcoming Migraines

The Vagus Nerve's Role in Migraine Pathogenesis

While trying to understand and get rid of headaches, we've looked into how the vagus nerve works and how it affects our health in a big way. Now, let's look at the interesting link between this nerve that wanders and headaches, which can be very painful and make it hard to do things. Researchers are still trying to figure out how migraines happen, but there is more and more proof that the vagus nerve plays a big part in how they start and maybe even how they go away.

The vagus nerve is an important piece in the puzzle of migraines.

An extensive network of fibers that reach into many parts of the body makes up the vagus nerve. It is an important communication link between the brain and many systems, including those that sense and control pain. If this connection is interrupted, it could be because of inflammation, stress, or something else. This can start a chain of events that lead to migraines' throbbing pain, nausea, and sensitivity to light and sound.

Researchers have found that people who get migraines often have less activity in their vagus nerve than people who don't get migraines. This decreased movement can make it harder for the body to control pain signals, which can make it more likely to experience the severe pain of migraines. The vagus nerve is also very important for controlling the release of chemicals like serotonin and dopamine, which help the brain deal with pain and keep its mood stable. Problems with the vagus nerve may cause these neurotransmitters to be out of balance, which may make headaches more likely to happen and get worse.

One thing that all inflammatory

More and more people are realizing that inflammation is a major cause of many long-term diseases, such as migraines. With its anti-inflammatory qualities, the vagus nerve naturally stops the body from having too much inflammation. This brake is released when the vagus nerve isn't working properly, which lets inflammation run wild and could cause or make headaches worse. Studies have shown that engaging the vagus nerve can lower inflammation and ease the pain of migraines, which makes this a potentially useful way to treat migraines.

The Link Between Gut and Brain

Another important part of migraine pathology that the vagus nerve plays is in the gut-brain axis, which is a network of nerves that communicate back and forth between the gut and the brain. The gut is home to trillions of microorganisms, which are all connected to each other and affect many body processes, such as the immune system, the production of neurotransmitters, and how we feel pain. Misbalances in the gut microbiome, which is also known as dysbiosis, have been connected to migraines and other brain illnesses.

Signals can travel from the gut to the brain through the vagus nerve. This lets the gut and brain talk to each other and change how each other works. Issues with this connection can lead to migraines, whether they are caused by gut dysbiosis, inflammation, or something else. On the other hand, probiotics and dietary changes that support a healthy gut bacteria may help ease migraine symptoms by balancing the gut-brain axis and improving vagus nerve function.

What Stress Does to the Vagus Nerve

Migraines are often caused by stress, and the vagus nerve is a key part of our body's reaction to stress. The sympathetic nervous system, which controls our "fight or flight" reaction, is activated when we are stressed, while the parasympathetic nervous system, which encourages rest and relaxation, is turned off. Along with other nerves in the parasympathetic nervous system, the vagus nerve is very important for keeping you calm and reducing the effects of worry.

Stress that lasts for a long time can damage the vagus nerve, making it less able to control stress hormones and help you rest. This imbalance can make us more likely to get headaches, which are very painful and uncomfortable. On the other hand, deep breathing exercises, meditation, and yoga can help lower stress and lessen the effects of migraine causes by increasing the activity of the vagus nerve.

Using Vagus Nerve Stimulation to Give Yourself Power Even though the vagus nerve's part in migraine pathogenesis may seem complicated, knowing this link gives us the power to manage and get rid of headaches. We can improve the function of our vagus nerve and keep our bodies in balance by making changes to our lifestyles, learning how to deal with stress, and getting focused therapies.

Vagus nerve stimulation (VNS) is a treatment method that involves sending electrical impulses to the vagus nerve. It has shown promise in helping people with migraines and other neurological problems. VNS can be given through implantable devices or non-invasive methods, like transcutaneous VNS (tVNS), which stimulates the vagus nerve through the skin. People who suffer from headaches may find relief in these treatments because they may reduce inflammation, change pain signals, and bring the nervous system back into balance.

Besides VNS, there are a few other ways to improve the function of the vagus nerve and maybe even ease the pain of migraines. The vagus nerve can be stimulated and relaxation can happen through deep breathing techniques, especially those that focus on slow, rhythmic exhalations. Meditation, yoga, and practicing awareness can also increase the activity of the vagus nerve and lower stress, which can help reduce the things that cause migraines.

Eating foods that are high in omega-3 fatty acids, probiotics, and anti-inflammatory substances can help keep the gut bacteria healthy and the vagus nerve working well. Also, staying away from processed foods, sugary drinks, and too much caffeine can help lower inflammation and keep blood sugar levels stable, which is good for the vagus nerve and may help reduce the number and intensity of migraines.

We can take back control of our health and well-being by focusing on the whole person and addressing the root reasons of migraines, such as vagus nerve dysfunction, inflammation, gut dysbiosis, and stress. Remember that getting rid of headaches isn't just about putting off the symptoms; it's also about supporting your body's natural ability to heal and recover. Thanks to its wide-ranging effects, the vagus nerve is a useful tool on this path that can help us live a life without headaches and full of health and happiness.

Vagus Nerve Stimulation to Treat and Prevent Migraines

When you have one of the millions of headaches that happen every year, you know how painful and annoying they can be. The headache, the sensitivity to light and sound, and the feeling of being sick... You might feel helpless because it's a vicious circle. But what if I told you there was a natural way to break out of this loop that wouldn't hurt you? As a result, vagus nerve stimulation (VNS) has become a revolutionary treatment that is changing how we avoid and treat migraines.

The Vagus Nerve is like a superhighway for your body. Before we can talk about how VNS works, we need to talk about the vagus nerve. This amazing nerve forms the superhighway of your body, linking your brain to many systems, such as your heart, lungs, and gut. It is a very important part of controlling many body processes, such as your stress response, heart rate, digestion, and even your migraines.

Researchers think that headaches might be caused by an imbalance in the activity of the vagus nerve. This nerve can set off a chain of events that lead to a migraine attack when it's not working right.

This is where VNS comes in. By gently stimulating the vagus nerve, we can help it get back to normal and maybe even lessen the number and severity of headaches.

How Stimulating the Vagus Nerve Works

There are a few different ways to send small electrical signals to the vagus nerve, which is how VNS works. One way is to have a small device surgically implanted under your chest skin. This device sends messages to the vagus nerve. People with severe migraines who haven't reacted to other treatments are usually the only ones who can get this.

But a type of VNS that doesn't hurt the person is also becoming more popular. To do this, you put a handheld device on your neck and use it to trigger the vagus nerve through your skin. You can do this at home, and most people think it's safe and okay.

How Vagus Nerve Stimulation Can Help with Migraines

What can VNS do to help your headaches? Studies have shown that the treatments are working, and many people have seen a big drop in how often and how bad their attacks are. Some people say that VNS can even stop headaches in their tracks.

But that's not the end of the good things. VNS has also been shown to boost happiness, lower anxiety, and make people healthier in general. This is because the vagus nerve controls how you feel and react to worry. We can help people feel calmer and more relaxed by stimulating this nerve. This can be very helpful for people with headaches who often feel very stressed and anxious.

Vagus Nerve Stimulation in Real Life: How It Works Here are some cases from real life that show how VNS has helped people get rid of migraines. Sarah, a 35-year-old woman who had been dealing with painful migraines for many years, got relief with non-invasive VNS. After only a few weeks of using the handheld device, she realized that her migraines happened much less often and were not as bad. She was also able to handle her stress better and feel like she had more power over her life.

John, a 42-year-old man who had tried many medicines and treatments but didn't get better, also turned to VNS. He chose to have the device implanted and was blown away by the effects. It not only made his migraines less common and less painful, but it also made his mood and quality of life much better overall.

Using your body's natural ability to heal itself Stimulating the vagus nerve is a strong method that can help your body heal itself and get rid of your migraines. It's a natural, painless way to get your nerve system back in balance, feel better overall, and lessen pain. If you're sick of living in fear of your next migraine, VNS might be the answer you've been looking for. Check with your doctor to make sure it's okay for you. It might help you get your life back and live without pain. Don't forget that you have help in this fight. You can get rid of your headaches and do well if you get the right tools and help.

Case studies and stories of success

When it comes to healing the vagus nerve, nothing works as well as real-life stories of people who beat headaches. Not just stories; these people are real proof that stimulating the vagus nerve can make a big difference. They give you hope, ideas, and a way to start your own healing process.

Emily is a woman in her mid-40s who has had terrible headaches for more than ten years. Every flare-up was like a storm in her head that kept her from doing anything for days. She tried many medicines, treatments, and changes to her lifestyle, but nothing worked. Emily was desperate for relief, so she looked into vagus nerve stimulation.

Emily began with easy routines like deep breathing and humming, which were suggested by her doctor. With the help of cold baths and yoga, she started doing these things every day. She was shocked when the number and severity of her headaches started to go down. It was getting less common and not as bad for the storms in her head.

Emily chose to try a non-invasive vagus nerve stimulator because she felt good about her progress. This hand-held device sent mild electrical signals to her vagus nerve, which made it work even better. The effects were truly amazing. This made her migraines even less common, and she also felt better in terms of her mood, energy, and general health. We can learn from Emily's experience that vagus nerve stimulation can help people who get headaches.

Moving on, let's talk about Michael, a young man who had headaches all the time since he was a teenager. Stress, bright lights, and some foods would often give him headaches. He had tried many medicines, but the side effects were often too much to handle. He felt like he was stuck in a loop of pain and anger.

Michael was told by a friend about vagus nerve stimulation and chose to try it. He began with easy things like meditation and deep breathing. He also tried changing what he ate, getting rid of foods that might have been triggers. He slowly began to notice a change. His headaches were happening less often and weren't as bad. He felt like he had more power over his life and body.

Michael chose to take his healing of the vagus nerve one step further after seeing how far he had come. He started going to a yoga class that was all about being aware and lowering stress. He also looked into acupuncture, which is known to activate the vagus nerve. Using all of these methods together made a huge difference in his migraines. He had fewer flare-ups, and the ones that did happen were much easier to deal with. Michael's story shows how important it is to heal the vagus nerve in a complete way, using a variety of ways to get the best results.

But vagus nerve stimulation isn't just for people who have had headaches for a long time. It can also help people who get migraines or headaches every once in a while. For example, Sarah was a woman in her early 30s who got migraines a few times a month. These headaches were generally caused by changes in her hormones or stress. Since she didn't want to take medicine, she chose to look into natural treatments.

Sarah learned about vagus nerve stimulation on the Internet and chose to give it a try. She began by doing easy things like gargling and singing. She also took cold showers every day and practiced deep breathing whenever she thought she might get a headache. She was surprised that these easy skills were enough to stop most of her headaches. She didn't have as bad of a headache when she did get one. Sarah's story shows that even simple techniques for stimulating the vagus nerve can help with occasional headaches.

In the world of vagus nerve healing, these are just a few of the many success stories that occur. What ties all of these stories together is the power of vagus nerve stimulation to change people's lives. Vasgus nerve stimulation could be the key to getting your body to fix itself, even if you've only had headaches once in a while or have had migraines for years.

Don't forget that these are just personal stories. What works for one person might not work for another of them. The important thing is to try out different methods until you find one that works for you. As you start your own healing journey for your vagus nerve, keep these stories in mind.

Allow them to give you hope, drive, and support. Your body can fix itself on its own, and vagus nerve stimulation can help you use that power.

Chapter 8: Conquering Anxiety and Depression

The Vagus Nerve and the Stress Response

Think of your vagus nerve as an old wise man who talks to your body and mind in a soothing way. As the leader of your parasympathetic nervous system, which is the "rest and digest" branch, it fights the "fight or flight" reaction that your sympathetic nervous system sets up. This powerful duo works together to keep a fine balance, like a seesaw that swings back and forth between calm and tense.

Stress in all its forms can throw off this balance and make your sympathetic nerve system work too hard. As you get ready to face a threat, your muscles lock up, your heart beats faster, and your breath quickens. In an emergency, this reaction can save your life, but long-term stress is bad for your health and can lead to anxiety, depression, and many other illnesses.

The vagus nerve is that part of your body that helps you deal with worry. It releases a chain reaction of calming chemicals, such as acetylcholine and GABA, when it is stimulated. These chemicals can stop your racing heart, slow your breathing, and rest your muscles. Picture a kind hand on your shoulder letting you know everything is okay.

Higher vagal tone, which is a measure of how active the vagus nerve is, makes people less likely to get anxious or depressed and more able to handle stress. For them, life's problems are like waves that they can ride with grace and ease. People with lower vagal tone, on the other hand, may find it hard to deal with worry and feel overwhelmed and worn out.

Well, the good news is that you can train your vagus nerve to work better, just like an athlete. You can make your parasympathetic nervous system stronger and better able to handle stress by doing things that activate the vagus nerve. Having a better sense of well-being can then lower your risk of anxiety and sadness.

Breathing deeply and slowly is one of the easiest and most effective ways to wake up your vagus nerve. Your diaphragm closes when you take a deep breath in, which stimulates the vagus nerve. Your heart rate slows down and your body rests as you slowly let out air. Just do this for a short time every day, and you'll be amazed at how quickly you can go from being stressed to being calm.

Humming or singing is another powerful way to stimulate the vagus nerve. These sounds make movements that connect with your vagus nerve and make it work to calm you down. Hit a favorite tune or say a word or phrase over and over, like "om" or "peace." For a double dose of vagus nerve activation, you can hum and take deep breaths at the same time.

If you splash cold water on your face or take a cold shower, you can also stimulate your vagus nerve. Even though it doesn't sound good, being cold can wake up your parasympathetic nervous system and help you rest and reduce inflammation.

Besides these methods, doing things that make you happy and connect with others can also help your vagal tone. Feel-good chemicals like oxytocin and dopamine can be released when you laugh, play, spend time with loved ones, or do artistic things. This can make your vagus nerve activity even stronger.

You can use the power of your vagus nerve to fight stress, anxiety, and sadness by making these adjustments to your daily life. Don't forget that your vagus nerve can help you become calmer, happy, and stronger. The vagus nerve has the power to change your life, but it takes work and time to fully   unlock   its   potential.

Helping with anxiety and depression through the vagus nerve

Anxiety and sadness are two of the most common mental health problems people have today, and they affect a huge number of people. The vagus nerve, on the other hand, is a sign of hope that is right inside us. This amazing nerve is like a superhighway for the brain and the rest of the body to talk to each other. It controls our mood, stress response, and general health. When we use the vagus nerve's power, we can find many natural, self-healing ways to help people who are anxious or depressed feel better, leading to a happier, brighter life.

The soothing embrace of the vagus nerve

Think of the vagus nerve as a gentle hand that eases your worries and makes you feel better. Neurotransmitters like acetylcholine and GABA are released when it is triggered.

These chemicals help to calm the mind, ease tension, and promote a sense of inner peace. This "vagal brake" balances out the stress reaction and helps you relax and deal with stress better. However, how can we trigger this strong nerve and use its healing power?

Every time you breathe, you release stress.

Being aware of your breathing is one of the easiest and most effective ways to wake up the vagus nerve. The vagus nerve gets signals to slow down the stress reaction and help you relax when you take deep, slow breaths, especially ones that focus on exhalation. It's kind of like a short break for your nervous system. Diaphragmatic breathing, also known as "belly breathing," alternate nostril breathing, and box breathing (equal counts for inhale, hold, exhale, hold) are all things you can try. Mindful breathing for just a few minutes can have a huge effect on your stress and happiness.

Being in the cold is a shock to the system (in a good way!). Strangely enough, being outside in the cold can be good for your vagal tone, even though it might not make sense. The vagus nerve is activated when you put your face in cold water or take a cold shower. This sets off a chain of physiological responses that can lower inflammation, improve mood, and make you more resistant to stress. If you've never been in the cold before, start slowly and build up to longer periods of time. You might be shocked at how energized and renewed you feel afterward.

As the saying goes, "music for the soul" (and the vagus nerve).

The voice cords, muscles in the throat, and the inner ear are all connected to the vagus nerve. These muscles are activated when we sing, hum, or pray. This then makes the vagus nerve work. This can make you feel calm, less anxious, and better about your mood. Your voice can heal your nervous system in powerful ways, whether you're singing your favorite songs in the shower or joining a band.

Meditation and mindfulness: training the mind and taming anxiety

Focusing on the current moment without judging it is a part of mindfulness and meditation. These practices have been shown to strengthen vagal tone and lower anxiety. We can learn to deal with stress in a more calm and aware way by becoming more aware of our thoughts and feelings. Regular meditating can change the way the brain works, which can help people control their emotions and be stronger. It can make a big difference in your health to do even a few minutes of mindful meditation every day.

Making friends is the vagus nerve's secret weapon. Self-care isn't the only thing the vagus nerve does; it's also very important for how we deal with others. Being around good people, talking, spending time with loved ones, and doing nice things for others can stimulate the vagus nerve and make us feel better. Strong social bonds may help protect against anxiety and sadness, which shows how important it is to take care of our relationships.

You can use your body's natural ability to heal and grow by incorporating these nerve interventions into your daily life.

Don't forget that it's a trip, not a race. Try out different methods and be patient with yourself as you find the ones that work best for you. As you work to improve your vagal tone, you'll open up a world of self-healing options and make life better and happier in the future.

Using Vagus Nerve Stimulation along with other treatments

When it comes to healing, vagus nerve stimulation is like a powerful song. But just like one instrument rarely plays a whole piece, vagus nerve stimulation can work even better when combined with other treatments. Think of it as a team effort, where each therapy brings its own skills to the table to make everyone feel better. This method takes into account how mind and body are linked and uses multiple pathways to help your body heal itself naturally.

How Vagus Nerve Stimulation and Therapy Work Together

Brain stimulation of the vagus nerve and therapy are two of the most hopeful combinations, especially for people who are dealing with anxiety and depression. Think of psychotherapy as a gentle guide who helps you find your way through the maze of your feelings and thoughts. On the other hand, stimulating the vagus nerve works like a helping hand, calming the physiological storms that often come with these conditions. According to research, this combined method may make both therapies work better, which could lead to fewer symptoms and better health in general.

Stimulation of the vagus nerve and mind-body practices

Another idea that should be looked into is how vagus nerve treatment can be combined with mind-body practices like yoga, meditation, and deep breathing. People have known for a long time that these practices can calm the nervous system and bring about mental peace. By adding vagus nerve stimulation, you may be able to boost their affects and create a relaxing symphony that goes through your body and mind. Imagine yourself in a relaxing yoga pose, your breath going smoothly, and the sound of your vagus nerve being stimulated adding to the experience. Together, they are very strong and can make you feel grounded, focused, and deeply at peace.

Nutritional therapies and stimulation of the vagus nerve
What you eat can even affect how well vagus nerve stimulation works for you. Eating a lot of anti-inflammatory foods, omega-3 fatty acids, and prebiotics can help your gut microbiome grow, which can then improve the health of your vagus nerve. It's like giving your nervous system the building blocks it needs to stay fit. When you stimulate the vagus nerve and eat well, you're basically making a perfect environment for repair and health   to   grow.

Stimulating the vagus nerve and physical therapy
In the field of physical rehabilitation, vagus nerve stimulation and physical training have been shown to work well together. This combined method might improve motor function and encourage neuroplasticity in people who are recovering from a stroke or other neurological problem.

Think of vagus nerve stimulation as a spark that gets the nervous system ready for the good changes that physical therapy is meant to bring about. This partnership has the ability to help people recover in new ways and feel like they have power again.

Making your healing journey unique

The great thing about vagus nerve stimulation is that it can be used with a lot of different treatments. You can't use the same method for everyone. Instead, it's about making a treatment plan that fits your specific goals and wants. Your doctor or nurse can help you through the process and help you choose the treatments that work best for you.

Remember that getting better is a run, not a sprint. To do it, you need to be patient, persistent, and open to trying new things. When you use vagus nerve stimulation along with other complementary treatments as part of a holistic approach, you're not only treating the symptoms but also getting to the bottom of your problems.

You're listening to your body's natural knowledge and giving yourself the power to make your life full of health, happiness, and vitality.

Chapter 9: Healing from Trauma

Trauma's Impact on the Nervous System

No matter if it's a single event that changes our lives or a number of smaller, ongoing stresses, trauma always leaves a mark on our nervous system. These events have a huge impact on this complex web of nerves that controls everything from our heartbeat to our emotions. A big part of getting better is understanding how stress affects our nervous systems.

Think of your nervous system as an orchestra, with each section playing its part perfectly in sync with the others. Trauma breaks up this harmony and makes it chaotic. It's like the fight-or-flight reaction, which is meant to keep us safe from harm, gets stuck in overdrive. Even when there is no threat, this state of hyperarousal puts us on high alert.

The amygdala, which is the brain's alarm system, becomes very busy and is always looking for danger. It pushes aside the prefrontal cortex, which is in charge of logical thought and making decisions. As a result, people feel more fear and worry, have trouble focusing, and act without thinking.

The vagus nerve, which is in charge of the parasympathetic nervous system, can also be damaged by long-term worry and trauma. As a brake, this nerve slows down the heart rate, clears the thoughts, and helps you relax. The vagus nerve gets weaker after trauma, which makes it harder to recover from stress and makes us more likely to have anxiety, sadness, and other health problems.

The good news is that our nerve system is very strong. In the same way that trauma can upset its balance, healing techniques can bring it back. Once we know how trauma changes the nervous system, we can make sure that our mending methods target the specific imbalances that trauma   causes.
Somatic treatments, which focus on the link between the body and mind, are one of the best ways to heal from trauma. These therapies help us get in touch with our bodies again, let go of feelings that are holding us back, and keep our nervous systems in balance. Yoga, meditation, and breathwork are some other techniques that can be very helpful for relaxing and calming the nervous system.

Remember that getting better after a traumatic event is a process, not a goal. You will face problems and failures along the way, but you can get your health and well-being back with patience, persistence, and the right help. You can come out of the darkness of pain stronger and more resilient than ever, just like a butterfly does when it comes out   of   its   chrysalis.
Making friends and family is another strong way to heal from trauma. People who have been through trauma often feel alone and shut down, but connecting with others can be very helpful. Telling someone you trust about your feelings or seeing a therapist can help you work through them and feel less alone. Doing things you enjoy with people you care about can also improve your mood and make you feel like   you   fit.
Food and exercise are also very important for getting better

after a traumatic event. A healthy, nutrient-dense food can help your nervous system stay healthy and heal. Getting regular exercise, like a brisk walk, yoga class, or dance class, can help relieve stress, boost happiness, and make you stronger.

Trauma can also make it hard to sleep, which can make us tired and irritated. Setting a regular sleep plan, making a relaxing bedtime routine, and staying away from screens before bed can all help improve the quality of your sleep and support your overall healing. It is important to know that there is no one way to heal from trauma that works for everyone.

Some people may not be able to use something that works for someone else. It's important to pay attention to your body, accept what it needs, and find the help that works for you.

Please don't be afraid to ask for help if you're having trouble with the effects of stress. Therapists, support groups, and online communities are just a few of the tools that are out there. You don' need to handle this by yourself. Don't forget that healing is possible. You can get over the problems caused by stress and live a full, happy life if you get the right help and tools. We are very strong and resilient on the inside, just like the vagus nerve is very important for our bodies to heal. We can get through hard times and come out better than ever if we use these tools.

We'll talk more about how awareness and meditation can help you heal from trauma in the next chapter. These activities can help us get to know ourselves better, keep our feelings in check, and find peace within.

The vagus nerve, which is like a superhighway for our bodies' information, is very important for healing from stress. It's the link between our mind and body, and it can become weak after a traumatic event. But knowing what the vagus nerve does can help us get better and take back our lives.

The Vagus Nerve and How We Respond to Trauma
The vagus nerve is like the director of the stress orchestra in your body. The "fight-or-flight" reaction is set off by the sympathetic nervous system when there is danger. This is a defense system that helps us stay alive and keep us safe. But when there is stress, the vagus nerve can get stuck in this state of high alertness, which can cause a chain reaction of physical and emotional symptoms.

PTSD can show up in our bodies in many ways, such as anxiety, panic attacks, sleeplessness, chronic pain, and digestive problems. The vagus nerve can do more than just scare us, though. It can also calm us down. It can start the "rest-and-digest" reaction, which makes you feel calm and relaxed, by activating the parasympathetic nervous system.

Polyvagal Theory and Healing from Trauma

The new and important Polyvagal Theory gives us even more information about how the vagus nerve helps us heal from trauma. The ventral vagal complex, also known as the "smart" vagus, and the dorsal vagal complex, also known as the "primitive" vagus, are thought to be the nerve's two sections.

The ventral vagal complex is in charge of making connections and interacting with other people. This branch is turned on when we feel safe and loved, which makes us feel good and strong. The dorsal vagal complex can take over, though, if trauma breaks this link. This can make you feel shut down and disconnected. To heal from trauma, it's important to understand this relationship. We can make ourselves feel safe even when our feelings are too strong by learning to use the ventral vagal complex. This helps us deal with stress and move on with our lives.

Vagus Nerve Stimulation: A Strong Way to Heal After a Trauma

Vasopressor stimulation (VNS) has become an interesting way to treat trauma-related illnesses like post-traumatic stress disorder (PTSD). Sending mild electrical signals to the vagus nerve is what VNS does. This helps to control its activity and speed up the healing process.

Studies have shown that VNS can help a lot with PTSD symptoms like dreams, flashbacks, and being too alert. It may also help with sleep, happiness, and living a better life in general. A healthcare worker is usually the one who does VNS, but there are easy things you can do at home to stimulate your vagus nerve.

How to Stimulate Your Vagus Nerve in Real Life

There are a few simple and successful ways to use your vagus nerve to heal yourself:

• Deep breathing: Taking slow, deep breaths calms your mind and body by activating the parasympathetic nervous system.

• Humming or singing: These activities make sounds that make the vagus nerve more active. The vagus nerve can be stimulated by splashing cold water on your face or taking a cold shower for a short time. This can improve your happiness.

• Social Connection: Your ventral vagal complex can get stronger when you spend time with people you care about, laugh, and have deep talks.

Mindfulness and meditation can help you better control your nervous system by making you more aware of how your body feels and what feelings it is experiencing.

Remember that it takes time and patience to heal from pain. But if you do these things every day, you can eventually make your vagus nerve stronger and feel better throughout the day.

What Happens When the Vagus Nerve Heals

The vagus nerve is not only a way to feel pain, but also a way to heal. By taking care of this link, we can help our bodies naturally heal and grow. As you start to heal, keep in mind that every little thing you do to improve the health of your vagus nerve affects the rest of your body.

Little things you do for yourself can make big changes in your body and mind, just like a butterfly moving its wings can cause a storm on the other side of the world. Accept the vagus nerve's power, and see how it changes your life in ways you never thought possible. The vagus nerve can help you heal from trauma. You can change the ending of your story and make a future full of peace, joy, and strength by understanding its role and using its healing power.

Don't forget that you're not going through this trip by yourself. Ask for help, be kind to yourself, and trust that your body's natural knowledge will lead you to healing.

Using the vagus nerve to help with trauma therapy Trauma is a fact of life for many people that can leave deep wounds in the mind and body. But, as we've seen, the vagus nerve, which is connected to many organs and systems in a complex way, may help people heal from stress. Today, we're going to talk about how vagus nerve-based methods can be revolutionary in trauma therapy.

How the body reacts to trauma and the vagus nerve The fight-or-flight reaction is a survival mechanism that our bodies automatically activate when we are faced with a traumatic event. It causes a surge of stress hormones. In times of immediate danger, this reaction is helpful, but activation that lasts too long or happens too often can mess up the vagus nerve and make PTSD and other trauma-related conditions worse.

You can change the vagus nerve's out of whack state, which is good news. It has amazing neuroplasticity, which means it can change how it works and reshape itself. Approaches that use the vagus nerve try to use this flexibility to bring balance back and help people heal from stress.

Therapy for trauma and polyvagal theory

Polyvagal theory, which was created by Dr. Stephen Porges, has changed the way we think about the vagus nerve's role in pain. It says that the vagus nerve has two separate branches: the ventral vagal complex is linked to social interaction and relationship, and the dorsal vagal complex is linked to shutting down and staying still. When these branches don't work properly because of trauma, the body relies too much on the dorsal vagal reaction. This can show up as mental numbness, withdrawing from others, and having trouble controlling your feelings. Based on polyvagal theory, methods that use the vagus nerve try to restore a sense of safety and encourage activation of the ventral vagal response.

Stimulation of the vagus nerve

Vagus nerve stimulation, or VNS, is a way to treat pain by sending small electrical signals to the vagus nerve. VNS has been used for a long time to treat epilepsy and depression, but new study shows that it may also help with symptoms related to trauma.

Researchers have found that VNS can lower hyperarousal, which is a sign of PTSD, and make it easier for the brain to process and integrate painful memories. By changing the activity of the vagus nerve, VNS may cause a state of physiological calmness and emotional regulation, which can help the body heal.

Stress and Breathing Exercises

A simple but effective way to stimulate the vagus nerve and help you relax is to breathe deeply and slowly. The parasympathetic branch of the vagus nerve is activated when we take deep breaths. This stops the stress reaction and makes us feel calm. People who have been through trauma often breathe quickly and shallowly, which is a sign of being highly alert. By doing deep breathing exercises, people can retrain their nervous systems to be more resilient in the face of stress and lessen the severity of symptoms linked to trauma.

Being Mindful and Trauma

Mindfulness, the practice of being aware of the present moment without judging it, has become an important part of trauma treatment. Mindful awareness training can help people feel more in charge of their feelings and thoughts, which can make upsetting memories less painful.

Mindfulness techniques, like body scans and meditation, can also raise vagal tone, which is a measure of how active the vagus nerve is. Having more vagal tone is linked to better emotional control, stress resilience, and general health.

Yoga and Hard Times

Yoga is a mind-body practice that includes meditation, breathing movements, and different body positions. It can help people heal from trauma in many different ways. According to research, yoga may help people with PTSD feel less anxious, depressed, and hyperaroused.

Yoga's gentle moves and stretches can help your body release tension. Focusing on your breath and being aware can help you relax and keep your emotions in check. By stimulating the vagus nerve and the parasympathetic nervous system, yoga can help you feel safe and at peace with yourself.

How Important It Is to Connect

Having been through trauma can make you feel alone and disconnected. Still, connecting with other people is a basic human need and a key part of the rebuilding process. By making friends and having important conversations, people can activate the ventral vagal complex, which makes them feel safe and like they belong. Group therapy, support groups, and community events can give people who have been through trauma a safe place to talk about their feelings, make new friends, and get stronger. By helping people bond with each other, we use the vagus nerve's natural ability to heal and restore.

The Way to Get Better

The way to get better after a traumatic event is very unique. Approaches that are built on the vagus nerve give people a wide range of tools to help them through this journey, giving them the tools they need to take back their lives and thrive. We can make the future better by using the power of the vagus nerve to help our bodies heal themselves.

Chapter 10: Addressing Other Chronic Conditions

Vagus Nerve Implications for Gut Health, Heart Health, Inflammation, and More

We've talked about the vagus nerve's role in a number of long-term diseases in this chapter. We've seen how it can help with headaches, stress, sadness, and long-term pain. But the vagus nerve affects a lot more than these usual health problems. It's an important part of staying healthy and happy all around, and it has big effects on gut health, heart health, inflammation, and more. Our gut, which is sometimes called our "second brain," is very closely linked to the vagus nerve. The gut and the brain talk to each other through this nerve. It sends signals back and forth that affect food, mood, and even immune function. The vagus nerve aids in digestion, intake of nutrients, and elimination of waste by maintaining a healthy gut environment when it is working at its best. It also helps keep the gut moving normally, which stops problems like diarrhea and constipation.

A strong link has been found between the vagus nerve and gut problems like irritable bowel syndrome (IBS). People with IBS often have less action in their vagus nerve, which makes their guts work less well and makes them more sensitive to pain. We can improve gut health, lower inflammation, and ease IBS symptoms by activating the vagus nerve.

The vagus nerve has a big effect on heart health as well. It is very important for keeping the heart rate and blood pressure in check, which helps keep the beat steady and stops arrhythmias. Studies have shown that people whose vagus nerves are more active tend to have healthier hearts and lower heart rates at rest. Low vagus nerve activity, on the other hand, has been linked to a higher chance of heart disease, stroke, and even sudden cardiac death.

One way the vagus nerve keeps the heart safe is by lowering swelling. Cardiovascular disease is made worse by chronic inflammation, which damages blood vessels and makes plaque build up. And because it reduces inflammation, the vagus nerve can help lessen this damage and keep the heart safe.

Whether it's short-term or long-term, inflammation is a normal reaction to injury or infection. Inflammation is necessary for healing, but too much or too long of it can do a lot of damage to the body and make a lot of long-term conditions worse, like autoimmune diseases, allergies, and even cancer. There is a nerve in the vagus body that helps control inflammation and keep it from getting out of hand.

When the vagus nerve detects inflammation, it tells the brain about it. The brain then releases chemicals that reduce inflammation and help the immune system calm down. This process, called the cholinergic anti-inflammatory pathway, is very good at lowering swelling and speeding up the healing process. We can use this pathway to help treat a number of inflammatory diseases by stimulating the vagus nerve.

The vagus nerve affects more than just inflammation, heart health, and gut health. A lot of other long-term illnesses have been linked to it, such as:

Research shows that stimulating the vagus nerve may help people who are overweight lose weight by making them feel fuller.

• Diabetes: The vagus nerve helps control blood sugar levels, and stimulating the vagus nerve has been shown to help people with diabetes better control their blood sugar levels.

Studies have shown that stimulating the vagus nerve may help slow the spread of Alzheimer's disease and make it easier to think and remember things. The possible benefits of stimulating the vagus nerve are very large and spread out. If we can use the power of this amazing nerve, we can help our bodies fix themselves and get rid of many long-term illnesses. If you are dealing with a long-term illness, I suggest that you look into the possible benefits of vagus nerve treatment. Talk to your doctor about this treatment to see if it might work for you. You can activate the vagus nerve in a number of ways, such as:

• Deep breathing exercises: Taking slow, deep breaths can help relax you by stimulating the vagus nerve.
• Doing yoga or meditating can help lower stress and make the vagus nerve work better.

• Singing and chanting: Singing and chanting can trigger the vagus nerve because they make vibrations.

It has been shown that acupuncture, an old technique, can make the vagus nerve work more.

• Massage: Some types of massage, like foot reflexology, can make the vagus nerve work better.
• Being in the cold for a short time, like when you take a cold shower or jump into a cold pool, can stimulate the vagus nerve.

Adding these things to your daily routine can help your vagus nerve get stronger and your health and well-being in general. Remember that the vagus nerve can help you get to the best health possible. By taking care of this nerve and using its full potential, you can help your body heal and grow naturally.

Customizing treatments for the vagus nerve for different conditions

Think of the vagus nerve as a director who leads your body's health like a symphony. But, just like in a symphony, each part needs a slightly different touch. Here, it's important to make sure that your vagus nerve treatments are right for you. You can tailor your vagus nerve exercises to fit your needs, just like a skilled tailor makes sure that a clothing fits perfectly.

Different Tools the Vagus Nerve Has

The vagus nerve is beautiful because it has many functions. There are many ways that it can help you because it affects many processes in your body. Let's look into how we can use this variety to heal specific areas.

Chronic Pain: Having chronic pain can make your life hard, but the vagus nerve can give you hope. Vagus nerve stimulation (VNS) may help change pain messages and lower inflammation, according to research. For rheumatoid arthritis and fibromyalgia, invasive VNS devices have shown promise. On the other hand, non-invasive ways such as transcutaneous auricular VNS (taVNS) are becoming more popular and easy to use.

But keep in mind that not all chronic pain is the same. If you have back pain, you might want to start with gentle routines that help you breathe deeply and move with awareness. If you have migraines, practicing relaxation methods like yoga or meditation could help calm down your nervous system.

Anxiety and Depression: The vagus nerve is very important for your mental health. Low vagal tone has been linked to more anxiety and sadness in studies. Luckily, you can make your vagal tone stronger by doing things like humming, praying, or taking deep breaths. These things make the vagus nerve work, which tells your brain to relax.

Think about this: when you take a deep, slow breath, you're rubbing your vagus nerve, which makes it send a wave of relaxation through your body. If your anxiety is getting the best of you, try mindfulness methods. By focusing on the present, you can break the circle of worry and make the vagus nerve calm down.

Digestive Problems: Did you know that your gut and the vagus nerve are closely linked? The gut-brain axis is another name for it. This link can help people who have stomach problems like irritable bowel syndrome (IBS). Deep belly breathing movements can help your body's digestion and ease pain in your gut by stimulating the vagus nerve.

Imagine that your breath is going all the way down to your stomach and massaging your intestines softly. Take this along with thoughtful eating habits like enjoying every bite and chewing it well. You will be taking care of both your gut and your vagus nerve at the same time.

Heart Health: Your vagus nerve is like a protection angel for your heart. It helps keep your blood pressure and heart rate in check, which is good for your heart health. To help this important function, do things that make you feel calm. The vagus nerve can be stimulated by yoga, tai chi, or even just being outside. This can help the heart relax and blood flow improve.
Think of your vagus nerve as a gentle hand that guides your heart to beat in a regular, relaxing way. You give your vagus nerve the tools it needs to keep your heart healthy by putting relaxation and stress relief first.

The Power of Customization: Research shows how useful the vagus nerve can be, but your trip is unique. What really helps one person might not help someone else at all. Allow yourself to try new things and find the solutions that work best for you.

You might find comfort in singing, or a warm bath might be the best way to stimulate your vagus nerve. The important thing is to pay attention to what your body is telling you and change your routines as needed.

A Lifelong Journey: Taking care of your vagus nerve isn't a quick fix; it's a journey of self-discovery and strength that lasts your whole life. Every time you take a deep breath, be mindful, or use a vagus nerve activation method, you help your body heal and grow naturally. Don't forget that you are in charge of your own health. One note at a time, you're writing a masterpiece of health by customizing your vagus nerve treatments.

Chapter 11: Maintaining a Healthy Vagus Nerve: Nurturing Your Body's Inner Superhighway

Excellent work! This article has helped you learn about the vagus nerve, how to activate it, and how it affects your health. Let us now talk about the long term: keeping the vagus nerve healthy. This isn't about a quick fix; it's about creating a way of life that helps this amazing nerve work at its best. Having a healthy vagus nerve doesn't just help with your current problems; it opens up a whole new level of well-being.

What the Vagus Nerve Eats Every Day: Lifestyle as Medicine

Think of the vagus nerve as a freeway that sends important messages all over your body. It needs regular upkeep to keep traffic moving smoothly, just like any other route. What does it look like to do this? It's surprisingly easy, and fun too!

• Get some exercise. Being active helps the vagus nerve. Moving around, whether you're taking a quick stroll in the park, doing yoga, or dancing in your living room, tells your brain that everything is fine. Try to do some kind of mild exercise most days of the week for at least 30 minutes.

• Deep Breaths: Do you remember the exercises you did to practice deep breathing earlier? They do more than just calm you down. The vagus nerve is stimulated by taking deep, slow breaths. This helps you relax and stay balanced. Do them every day.

• Sing, hum, or chant: It's true that the muscles used for singing and humming move the vagus nerve. Sing your favorite songs in the shower, join a band, or just hum a soft tune to yourself.

• Spend time with other people. Being around other people is good for your vagus nerve as well as your soul. Spend time with people you care about, have deep talks, and take care of your relationships. Laughter and good relationships with other people have a big effect on vagal tone.

• Cold Exposure: A short blast of cold water might not sound fun, but it's a great way to get the vagus nerve working. Finish your shower with a cold rinse, splash cold water on your face, or even go for a cold swim.

• Nutritious Foods: What you eat is very important for the health of your vagus nerve. Eat lots of fruits, veggies, whole grains, and healthy fats that have not been processed. Also good for you are the probiotics that are found in fermented foods like yogurt and pickles.

Mindfulness techniques, such as yoga and meditation, help calm the nervous system and make the vagus nerve stronger. Mindful breathing can help even for just a short time.

Care Plan for the Long Term for the Vagus Nerve

Along with your daily habits, here are some long-term tips for keeping your vagus nerve healthy:

• Dealing with stress: Long-term stress is bad for the vagus nerve. Deal with your stress in a healthy way, like by practicing mindfulness, going to therapy, or spending time in nature.

• Sleep Well: Getting enough sleep is important for your health in general, and this includes your vagus nerve. Aim to get at least 7-8 hours of good sleep every night. Regular Checkups: Make sure you get regular checkups with your doctor and take care of any underlying health problems that might affect the function of your vagus nerve.

• Think about supplements. Omega-3 fatty acids, magnesium, and probiotics are some substances that may help keep your vagus nerve healthy. Before you start taking any new vitamins, talk to your doctor.

Your health and the vagus nerve

Remember that keeping your vagus nerve healthy is a process, not a goal. It's about making choices every day that help this amazing nerve work at its best. As you take care of your vagus nerve, you'll be amazed at how much better you feel overall. You'll feel less stressed, have a better mood, handle food better, have less inflammation, and be stronger.

The vagus nerve runs through your body like a freeway.

t will give you a smoother, better ride through life if you take care of it.

Setting up a self-care routine that you can stick to: the basis for healing

We've looked at a lot of different techniques and treatments in our quest to understand and use the power of the vagus nerve. But the art of self-care is the most important thing that holds it all together. You can think of it as the good dirt where your vagus nerve and your whole body can grow.

Why taking care of yourself isn't selfish

Self-care is something that we often forget to do because our lives are so busy. We might think of it as a treat that we don't need or have time for. Okay, let's change that thought. Take care of yourself, but don't treat yourself like a princess. It means giving your mind and body the tools they need to heal, stay healthy, and grow. Self-care habits can have a big effect on our health, according to research. They can lower inflammation, lower stress chemicals, and make the vagus nerve work better. In turn, this can make migraines less common and less severe, improve your mood, and make you feel stronger.

The Things That Make Up Your Daily Schedule

Self-care isn't the same for everyone. Your journey is very important to you. But here are some important things you might want to think about as you make your routine:

Mindfulness and relaxation: Regular mindfulness meditation, deep breathing exercises, or even just a mindful walk in nature can help lower stress and start the parasympathetic reaction in the vagus nerve, which calms the body down.

• Moving: For healthy vagus nerves, it's important to do light exercise. As well as making you feel better, yoga, tai chi, and even dancing can help your health and circulation. Don't forget that the goal is to enjoy moving, not to push yourself too far.

• Sleep: Getting enough good sleep is important for recovery and healing. Aim for 7-8 hours of sleep each night and stick to a regular sleep routine to get the most out of your vagus nerve.

• Nutrition: Eat whole, raw foods that are good for your brain and body. A healthy diet full of vitamins, probiotics, and omega-3 fatty acids can help keep the vagus nerve healthy and lower inflammation.

• Connection: People need good connections in their lives because we are social animals. Spend time with people you care about, have deep talks, or think about joining a support group.

• Play and creativity: Give yourself time to discover your creative side or just do things you love. Painting, writing, gardening, or playing with your pet are all things that can help you feel better and less stressed.

Getting it to last

Making a self-care practice that you can stick to is important for its success. Start with a few simple things and add new ones over time. Be adaptable and ready to make changes when they're needed. Keep in mind that it's not about being great, but about getting better.

To keep you on track, here are some ideas:

• Make time for it: Schedule time for self-care like you would any other important meeting. Set aside time on your calendar and decide how important it is.

• Figure out what works for you. Try out different tasks until you find the ones that you enjoy the most.
• Don't be hard on yourself if you miss one or two days. You can just pick up where you left off.

Your power is taking care of yourself.

Taking care of yourself is an investment in your health and happiness. Taking care of your healing journey and making your life feel full and alive is a way to empower yourself.

Getting stronger and learning how to deal with stress Physical or mental situations that last for a long time can throw us curveballs and test how strong and resilient we are. They may have an effect on our general health, our relationships, and our daily lives. Even so, we can give ourselves the tools we need to not only survive but also grow. We can turn these problems into steps toward a more satisfying life by becoming more resilient and getting better at dealing with stress. Your inner strength is called resilience.

Being resilient is like having a mental shock absorber that helps you handle the ups and downs of life. It means being able to get back on your feet after something bad happens, deal with change, and keep your hope and positivity. It's not about denying or stifling hard feelings; it's about recognizing them, learning from them, and using them to drive your growth.

Increasing your resilience is an ongoing process that includes taking care of different parts of your health. Starting with taking care of your mind and body is important. You should make sure you get enough sleep, eat a healthy diet, and exercise regularly. These simple self-care habits can make it a lot easier for you to deal with problems and stress.

Having a good attitude is another important part of being resilient. To do this, you need to learn to be grateful, be kind to yourself, and fight bad thoughts. When you experience failures, think of them as chances to learn and grow. Remember that small wins can add up to a stronger sense of resilience over time.

Managing stress: How to Tame the Beast

Stress is a normal reaction to the things that happen in life, but too much of it can be bad for our mental and physical health. Stress that lasts for a long time can cause or make health problems worse, like migraines, anxiety, sadness, and other long-term pain problems. That's why learning how to deal with stress well is so important. Becoming more aware is one of the best ways to deal with stress. This means focusing on the present moment without judging it. You can become more mindful in many ways, such as through mindfulness meditation, yoga, and deep breathing techniques. These activities can help you feel better generally, calm your nervous system, and lower your stress.

Besides that, doing things you enjoy can also help you deal with stress. Find things that make you happy and make them a part of your daily life. This could be spending time in nature, listening to music, reading a book, or following a hobby. These things can give you a break from the worries of everyday life and help you feel better.

Putting together your tools

There is no one-size-fits-all answer to building resilience or dealing with stress. Some people may not be able to use something that works for someone else. It's important to try different things until you find what works for you. You might want to put together a collection of skills that you can use when things get tough. Here are some more useful tools for building resilience and dealing with stress:

• Make friends, family, or support groups to connect with.

Talking about your problems and getting support can be very inspiring.

• Therapy: Talking to a therapist can help you feel safe as you work through your feelings and find ways to deal with them.

• Writing in a journal: Writing down your thoughts and feelings can help you understand them better and deal with tough feelings.

• Creative Expression: Making art, music, or doing other creative things can help you deal with stress and worry. Remember that getting stronger and dealing with worry are ongoing processes. Along the way, there will be problems and failures, but don't give up. You can build the strength and resilience to not only get through hard times but also grow in them if you are patient, persistent, and have the right tools.

In the next part, we'll talk more about how to make sure you get the best care for your chronic conditions by being your own advocate and knowing how to use the healthcare system. Let's talk about how to talk to your healthcare workers in a way that gets your needs met and how to be an active part of your treatment plan.

It's easy to forget how important human connections are in a world where everything is linked. Still, feeling like we belong and having support is very important for our general health, especially when we are dealing with the challenges of long-term conditions. The vagus nerve has a butterfly effect that goes beyond our bodies and into our communities and social networks, building a strong web of support that can help us feel better and heal.

The Study of How to Help Others

A lot of research has shown that being socially connected is good for your mental and physical health. Strong social bonds have been shown to lower the chance of chronic diseases, boost the immune system, and even make people live longer. This is because oxytocin, which is sometimes called the "love hormone," is released when people connect with each other. Oxytocin lowers blood pressure, lowers stress, and makes people feel good.

A strong feeling of community and belonging can also protect against the bad effects of stress. A lot of long-term illnesses, like migraines, anxiety, and depression, can be made worse by long-term worry. Supportive groups can help people deal with the emotional and mental burdens of their conditions by giving them a safe place to talk about their experiences, let off steam, and get support.

Community as a Force for Change

In addition to offering emotional support, communities can also play a key role in encouraging people to make good changes to their lifestyles, which are necessary for managing chronic conditions. Whether it's a mindfulness meditation circle, a group exercise class, or a healthy cooking club, doing things with other people can give you a sense of accountability and motivation that you don't get when you're doing things by yourself.

Also, groups can provide a lot of information and help that can be very useful for people dealing with complicated chronic illnesses. Members can give each other the power to make smart choices about their health and well-being by sharing their experiences, thoughts, and tips. This shared knowledge can be especially helpful for people who feel alone or stressed out because of their condition.

How to Find Your Tribe

These days, thanks to technology, there are lots of ways to meet people with similar hobbies and experiences. Online support groups, social media boards, and forums are easy to join and provide a way to connect with others and build community. It's important to remember, though, that not every online community is the same. Look for groups that are moderated, have supportive members, and post messages that are upbeat and uplifting.

You could join a neighborhood support group, go to a community event, or do volunteer work for a cause you care about. You can meet new people, make connections that matter, and feel like you fit by doing these things. Don't forget that little things can make a big difference. A friendly smile, a kind word, or a helping hand can make someone's day better and spread happiness.

Putting together a helpful network

It takes time and work to build a strong support network, whether it's online or off. If you need help, don't be afraid to ask for it. Be patient with yourself and with other people. Remember that being open and honest is not a sign of weakness; it's a strength that can help people connect and trust each other more. As you work to build your group, pay attention to the energy you bring to the conversations you have. Communication that is positive, helpful, and encouraging can make everyone feel welcome and give them power. Honor each other's accomplishments, be there for each other when things get tough, and push each other to new heights.

What Connection Does to Others

When you open yourself up to the healing and support power of community and social relationship, you can change your life and the lives of those around you. Remember that the vagus nerve's butterfly effect isn't just about changing one person; it's about making a wave of well-being that can lift whole communities. So, connect with other people and let the world know about your light. We can all have a better, healthier, and more linked future if we work together.

Conclusion: Embrace the Ripple Effect - Summary of Key Takeaways

As we come to the end of our look at the vagus nerve and how it affects our health and well-being, let's go over the most important things you should remember to help your body heal itself and get over mental health problems and constant pain.

1. The vagus nerve is like the superhighway of your body. The vagus nerve is a very interesting way for your brain and body to talk to each other. It is very important for keeping your nervous system in check and can affect how you react to stress, how well your immune system works, how well your stomach works, and even how you feel. By knowing how powerful it is, you can use it to heal yourself.

2. Headaches, stress, sadness, and more: A problem with the vagus nerve is often linked to both long-term pain and mental health problems like sadness, anxiety, and migraines. You can ease your symptoms and make your life better in general by treating this underlying cause. Don't forget that you're not on this trip by yourself.

3. The Polyvagal Theory: A Different View: The polyvagal theory changes the way we think about the different parts of the vagus nerve and how they affect how we deal with stress and social situations. With this information, you can find your own vagal tone and make changes to your routines to improve the balance of your nervous system.

4. Stimulating the vagus nerve: a powerful tool Vagus nerve stimulation (VNS) techniques are a safe and successful way to heal by stimulating the vagus nerve. You can change VNS to fit your needs. It can be used for easy things like deep breathing and humming or for more complex things like yoga and meditation.

5. Making changes to your lifestyle: feeding your vagus nerve: The way you live is very important for the health of your vagus nerve. Creating an atmosphere that supports healthy vagus nerve function includes eating a balanced diet full of anti-inflammatory foods, working out regularly, making sleep a priority, and making friends who are positive influences.

6. The Mind-Body Link: Using Your Inner Strength: Your mind and body are one and the same. The way you think, feel, and believe can affect the function of your vagus nerve, which in turn affects your physical and mental health. Mindfulness practice, a good attitude, and doing things that make you happy can strengthen the mind-body connection and improve the function of the vagus nerve.

7. The Ripple Effect: How It Can Change Your Life: As you accept these important lessons and use them in your daily life, good things will start to happen all around you. You'll feel less pain, have better happiness, be able to handle stress better, and have a general sense of well-being. These changes will have an effect on your neighborhood, work, relationships, and life in general.

8. Enjoy the Journey: How to Get Better: Healing doesn't happen in a straight line. Remember to be kind to yourself as you go through the ups and downs. Enjoy your success, no matter how small it is, and don't give up on getting healthier. Your body can fix itself, and you can use the full power of that ability by using your vagus nerve.

This vagus nerve is more than just a nerve; it's an important part of your health. You can get rid of chronic pain and mental health problems and live a full, happy, and strong life by knowing how your body works, using strategies that have been shown to work, and taking a holistic approach to your health.

Always keep in mind that your situations do not define you. You are an amazing being with the power to heal and change. Let's embrace the ripple effect and start this fun trip of getting to know ourselves and being strong together.

You're now on a journey of learning, looking into how the vagus nerve affects your health in deep ways. The fact that you understand how it works and can use its power is a huge step toward healing and change. But, like any important journey, this one doesn't stop here.

Your vagus nerve trip is an ongoing adventure that lets you learn more about your body's natural ability to heal and grow. Taking care of your vagus nerve can have a chain reaction of good effects on your health and happiness, like how a butterfly's wings spread out and make waves of change.

You have a lot of potential locked up in the information you've learned. You can open it by practicing regularly and taking care of yourself. Whether you're doing deep breathing exercises, practicing awareness, or looking for ways to connect with other people, every small step you take is an important one for your health.

As you continue to connect more deeply with your vagus nerve, think of all the things that could happen. Imagine a life where migraines are a thing of the past, anxiety isn't as strong, and sadness gives way to newfound happiness. Imagine being calm and strong even when life throws you problems, knowing that you have the tools to get through any storm.

Stimulating the vagus nerve has been shown to improve mental health and chronic pain conditions in the long run. Studies show that stimulating the vagus nerve can lessen the number and severity of migraines, help people with anxiety and sadness feel better, and even speed up the healing process in people with chronic pain conditions like fibromyalgia.

As an example, Sarah, a woman who had terrible headaches for years, is very inspiring. Since she learned about the vagus nerve's power, she started doing exercises for it every day. Over time, she realized that her migraines happened much less often and were not as bad. She now feels like she has the power to take care of her health and live a pain-free life.

John's story is also very moving. He had anxiety and sadness for most of his life. He was stuck in a loop of sadness and negativity and couldn't get out of it. Being aware and doing exercises for the vagus nerve helped him when he learned about the link between it and mental health. He noticed a change in his mood and attitude over time. It made him feel better to be around and gave him more hope for the future.

These stories only show a small part of how the vagus nerve can change things. Don't forget that you are not alone as you go on your journey. More and more people are learning about the vagus nerve's possibilities and talking about their own experiences. Get to know other people, listen to their stories, and be inspired by their victories. Enjoy how your trip along the vagus nerve will affect other people. Help others heal by sharing what you know and encouraging them to do the same. Working together, we can make a world where being healthy is not just a dream, but a reality.

Don't forget that every trip starts with a single step. Every time you do something like deep breathing, mindfulness, or making friends, you are moving toward a healthier, happy you. Keep going, keep looking around, and keep thinking that your body has the power to heal itself. You can enjoy the butterfly effect of the vagus nerve.

Remember that there is no one-size-fits-all way to deal with your vagus nerve as you go along. Try out different methods until you find the one that works best for you. Be patient with yourself. The important thing is to be consistent and open to exploring your huge potential. So, I want you to keep learning, keep working, and keep telling other people about your journey. The vagus nerve's butterfly effect is a strong force for good. If you accept it, you can live a healthier, happier, and more fulfilling life.

Resources to Look into Further

Excellent work! This article has taken you on a trip through the vagus nerve and how it affects your health. By knowing how powerful it is, you've opened the door to a world of self-healing possibilities. But this is only the start. Your journey into the health of your vagus nerve can last a lifetime, full of new discoveries, personal growth, and better and better health. One of the best things about this trip is that it can be changed to fit your wants and interests. You can't use the same method for everyone. It's up to you to make this road your own. Use your curiosity and intuition to shape it. You'll find new techniques and ideas that really speak to you as you keep learning and trying new things. Don't forget that every little step forward is important.

Learning More About the Vagus Nerve

The field of vagus nerve study is always changing, and new findings are made all the time. By keeping up with the latest research, you can learn more about this interesting system and come up with new ways to use its power. There are many ways to keep up with the news:

• Books and articles: There is a lot of writing about the vagus nerve. Read books by professionals in the field, like Dr. Stephen Porges, who came up with the Polyvagal Theory, or Dr. Arielle Schwartz, who writes a lot about healing from trauma. A lot of trustworthy websites, like Psychology Today and the National Institutes of Health (NIH), also have articles about the newest study.

• Online Workshops and studies: The vagus nerve is covered in a lot of online workshops and studies. These can be a great way to get advice from experts and meet people who are interested in the same things you are.

• Scientific Journals: If you want to learn more, you might want to look into scientific journals that publish vagus nerve studies. You'll be able to read the newest research, even if the wording is more technical.

• Adding to Your Toolbox: Therapies and Methods Besides learning more about your condition, there are many other treatments and activities you can try to improve the health of your vagus nerve. Here are a few to get you going:

• Yoga and Tai Chi: These gentle forms of movement can help lower stress, make you more flexible, and calm you down, all of which are good for the vagus nerve.

Meditation and being aware: Regular meditation can raise

the tone of your vagus nerve and help you feel more calm and at peace with yourself.

• Deep breathing exercises: slow, deep breathing stimulates the vagus nerve, which leads to the relaxation reaction and lowers   stress.
• Sound therapy: Chanting, singing, or listening to soothing music are all sounds that can trigger the vagus nerve and help you relax.

Acupuncture and acupressure are forms of traditional

Chinese medicine that can help keep the body's energy in balance and make the vagus nerve work better.

Cold: Putting an ice pack on your neck or taking a cold shower for a short time can stimulate the vagus nerve and make you stronger.

Making friends in a community

Don't forget how important it is to have support in your healing process. Meeting people who are also interested in vagus nerve health can be a great way to get support, ideas, and knowledge.

Find support groups in your area, online, or on social media where you can share your stories and learn from others.

Taking a more complete look at things

Remember that the health of your vagus nerve isn't just about one or two methods or therapies. It's about taking a look at health from all angles.

• Take care of your body: For the vagus nerve to work at its best, you need to eat a healthy diet full of whole foods, exercise regularly, and make sleep a priority.

• Make friends and build relationships that matter. Having strong social ties and deep bonds can help you deal with stress and improve vagal tone.

• Do things you enjoy: Schedule time for hobbies, artistic projects, and other things that make you happy and satisfied. Having a feeling of purpose, laughing, and being playful are all good for your vagus nerve. The Effect of Ripples: Your journey goes on Remember that the vagus nerve is only one part of your health as you continue to learn and try new things.

When you take care of your vagus nerve, you not only make your own life better, but you also make the lives of those around you better.

When you're calm, strong, and caring, those traits easily come out in other people. Your health and happiness spread to everyone you meet, making them better. As you start this path of healing and self-discovery, keep in mind that you're not only changing your own life, you're also making the world healthier and happier.

The road ahead may have turns and twists, but you'll get through it with grace and courage if you use your interest as a compass and your strength as a guide. As you continue to learn and explore, remember to have faith in your body's natural ability to heal and grow. You are in charge of your own path to better vagus nerve health, and there are many options available.

www.ingramcontent.com/pod-product-compliance
Lightning Source LLC
Chambersburg PA
CBHW071024250726
48653CB00005B/1703